Clinical Guidelines in Old Age Psychiatry

Clinical Guidelines in Old Age Psychiatry

Alistair Burns MD FRCP FRCPsych MPhil
Professor of Old Age Psychiatry
University of Manchester
Manchester
UK

Tom Dening MA MD FRCPsych
Consultant Psychiatrist and Clinical Director
Psychiatric Services for the Elderly
Addenbrooke's NHS Trust, Cambridge and
Senior Professional Advisor
Department of Health, London
UK

Brian Lawlor MD FRCPI FRCPsych
Conolly Norman Professor of Old Age Psychiatry
Trinity College Dublin and
Consultant in Old Age Psychiatry
St Patrick's and St James's Hospitals
Dublin
Ireland

MARTIN DUNITZ

© Martin Dunitz Ltd 2002

First published in the United Kingdom in 2002 by

Martin Dunitz Ltd
The Livery House
7–9 Pratt Street
London NW1 0AE

Tel: +44-(0)20-7482-2202
Fax: +44-(0)20-7267-0159
E-mail: info.dunitz@tandf.co.uk
Website: http://www.dunitz.co.uk

A CIP catalogue record for this book is available from the British Library

ISBN 1-84184-029-7

Distributed in the USA by
Fulfilment Center
Taylor & Francis
7625 Empire Drive
Florence, KY 41042, USA
Toll Free Tel: 1-800-634-7064
Email: cserve@routledge ny.com

Distributed in Canada by
Taylor & Francis
74 Rolark Drive
Scarborough
Ontario M1R 4G2, Canada
Toll Free Tel: 1-877-226-2237
Email: tai fran@istar.ca

Distributed in the rest of the world by
ITPS Limited
Cheriton House
North Way, Andover
Hampshire SP10 5BE, UK
Tel: +44- (0)1264 332424
Email: reception@itps.co.uk

Composition by Wearset, Boldon, Tyne and Wear
Printed and bound in Italy by Legoprint.

Contents

Foreword

As the discipline of old age psychiatry develops throughout the world and as service delivery to older persons with mental disorders flourishes in many countries, the gaps in knowledge appear as chasms in the field. To fill these gaps of knowledge in the most "user-friendly" manner, Burns, Lawlor and Craig produced *Assessment Scales in Old Age Psychiatry* in 1999 providing a most useful and user-friendly compendium for all of us in the field of old age psychiatry.

Not resting in their well-earned laurels, Burns and Lawlor have, with the inclusion of Tom Dening, now produced the next most user-friendly compendium in *Clinical Guidelines in Old Age Psychiatry*, thus filling another gap for the front line workers who have to do the work and at the same time, satisfy policy makers and bureaucrats which demand, as the current fashion dictates, clinical pathways (guidelines), with expectation that those will provide outcomes to match the expectation of economic rationalistic penchants of the "bottom-line".

As psychiatry in general struggles with such demands, the authors quietly went about collating this volume of clinical guidelines for the old age psychiatrists in the field, thus doing another great service for us all.

Not content with such a collection, a labour of much effort, the authors have produced a masterful and intellectually vigorous Introduction, which serves to establish the essential issues in an honest and critical (in a positive sense) manner. This part of the volume is compulsory reading for all old age psychiatrists.

Once again, the world of old age psychiatry owes a debt of gratitude to Alistair Burns who produced the first edition of *Dementia* (Burns & Levy) and *Assessment Scales in Old Age Psychiatry* (Burns, Lawlor and Craig) has contributed greatly to the field. We should now also thank Tom Dening and Brian Lawlor who have joined with Alistair in this endeavour. We who are in the front-line of old age psychiatry salute you.

Edmond Chiu
Melbourne
June 2001

President, International Psychogeriatric Association
Chair, Old Age Psychiatry Section World Psychiatric Association

Preface

Old age psychiatry is unquestionably an area which is promising territory for the development of guidelines. There is a proliferation of information from various sources, but for the individual clinician it can be hard to find if suitable guidelines on a particular topic exist, since there is no comprehensive source with which to consult. Our aim is to bring as much of this material together so that the reader can obtain a view of the field and perhaps begin to form judgements about which guidelines are 'better' (be that better conceived, better constructed, better presented, more accessible, or easier to use).

In view of these considerations, we have used a broad conceptualization of 'guidelines' and included material that might be more accurately described by other terms, such as consensus statements or practice policies. In part, this is to portray the range of material and indicate the diversity of sources where guidance may be found lurking. However, the common theme of these sources seems to be that they provide direct advice to clinicians and others responsible for services with a view to achieving more standardized and consistent practice.

We have also presented material with a minimum of interpretation, partly to be consistent with a companion volume (Burns et al, 1999) where this approach has proved

successful, but partly to allow the reader to peruse and extract what they find helpful. The annotations are intended to be concise and descriptive. We hope that this presentation will enable readers to use the material to facilitate the development of their own guidelines or indicate where a more systematic approach is required to existing guidance.

This book, therefore, seeks to compile such guidance as exists in old age psychiatry. It is unlikely to be comprehensive but this may encourage readers to let us know what we have missed or else where no guidelines currently exist people may feel inspired to develop some!

Alistair Burns
Manchester
Tom Dening
Cambridge
Brian Lawlor
Dublin
June 2001

Reference

Burns A, Lawlor B, Craig S (1999) *Assessment Scales in Old Age Psychiatry*. London: Martin Dunitz.

Clinical Guidelines: An Introduction

Clinical guidelines have been defined as systematically developed statements which assist clinicians and patients in making decisions about appropriate treatment for specific conditions (NHS Executive, 1996).

Clinical guidelines are a growth area. For example, a recent Medline search produced almost 46 000 titles compared with 'only' 27 000 for 'Alzheimer's disease'. There is a sizeable literature on guidelines, their development, implementation and evaluation, so it is quite possible to develop guidelines upon guidelines! (Perhaps 'meta-guidelines' would be a suitable term.)

The terminology used is somewhat confusing in this area (Greenwood, 1999). *Consensus statements* may overlap with guidelines, the main difference being perhaps that consensus statements are not necessarily systematically derived. *Protocols* are written plans specifying the procedures to be followed in giving a particular examination or in providing care for a particular condition, so they have a narrower focus than guidelines. *Policies* are principles or statements that govern an activity and that employees of an institution are expected to follow, so a locally adapted guideline could fall under this heading, whereas most policies will certainly not be clinical guidelines. *Integrated care pathways* determine locally agreed, multidisciplinary practice, based on the best available evidence for a specific patient or client group. A care pathway forms all or part of the clinical record, documents the care given and facilitates the evaluation of outcomes. Thus a care pathway represents the application of a guideline in a practical situation.

Why have clinical guidelines?

The aim of having guidelines is to improve the quality of patient care. However, they form only a part of a wider effort to bring research findings into clinical practice. This wider aim is known as clinical effectiveness. The implementation of clinical guidelines may bring several benefits, including promoting evidence-based practice; supporting junior medical, nursing and other staff; supporting non-specialists; encouraging multidisciplinary working; and facilitating seamless care between different staff or different agencies.

To decide which areas may benefit most from having clinical guidelines, the NHS Executive (1996) publication on *Clinical Guidelines* suggests five criteria for deciding whether guidelines would be helpful:

1. where there is excessive morbidity, disability or mortality;
2. where treatment offers good potential for reducing morbidity, disability or mortality;
3. where there is wide variation in clinical practice around the country;
4. where the services involved are resource-intensive – either high volume and low cost or low volume and high cost;
5. and where there are many boundary issues involved, sometimes cutting across primary, secondary and community care, and sometimes across different professional bodies.

The conditions within the scope of old age psychiatry clearly meet all these requirements, so guidelines should play an important part in improving the quality of clinical services in old age psychiatry.

Constructing clinical guidelines

Often they originate from clinical groups with a special interest, or a professional body such as a Royal College, or a national or international organization. Sometimes there is a systematic initiative to produce a wide range of guidelines across medical specialities, for example the French Clinical Guidelines and Medical References programme (Maisonneuve *et al*, 1997).

To construct guidelines it is first necessary to decide which types of evidence are suitable. There are various ways to grade evidence from randomized controlled trials (RCTs) down to the statements of experts or received practice. Such systems include those used by the Agency for Healthcare Research and Quality (formerly the Agency for Health Care Policy and Research) (*www.achpr.gov*), the American Psychiatric Association and the Scottish Intercollegiate Guidelines Network (SIGN) (*www.show.scot.nhs.uk/sign*). A simple classification is that used by the NHS Clinical Outcomes Group:

(A) RCTs
(B) other robust experimental or observational studies
(C) more limited evidence but the evidence relies on expert opinion and has the endorsement of respected authorities.

Ideally, perhaps, guidelines should be developed following an initial systematic and critical review of the literature (Cook *et al*, 1997). However, in many areas of medicine the available evidence from RCTs and experimental studies is lacking so other methods involving the development of consensus are required (Trickey *et al*, 1998). This is true of the current state of much of old age psychiatry, for example the diagnosis and management of dementia. For other disorders, notably depression, older patients have often been excluded from studies or those that are included may not be typical of the general older population, so published findings may not be readily generalizable (Banerjee and Dickinson, 1997).

The content of guidelines should specify the patient population concerned, indicate the provenance of the evidence used, and set out the likely costs, benefits and implications of implementation. Successful guidelines should be valid, reproducible, reliable, cost-effective, representative, clinically applicable, flexible, clear, reviewable and amenable to audit (NHS Executive, 1996). Guidelines may be presented in a variety of forms for differing readerships, for example those of the National Guideline Clearinghouse (NGC) (*www.guideline.gov*).

Appraisal of guidelines

How can you tell if the guideline is valuable or useful? There are three approaches to the appraisal of guidelines, the first being an official appraisal which ordains whether a guideline should be used for official purposes, for example health care commissioning. In the UK, guidelines may be appraised by the NHS Appraisal Centre for Clinical Guidelines and may then be commended for use in health

commissioning by the NHS Executive. This appraisal will follow a standard approach (Cluzeau *et al*, 1997; see also *www.sghms.ac.uk/depts/phs/hceu/clinguid.htm*), but not all guidelines will be suitable for this consideration. The Clinical Outcomes Group also believes that only evidence from RCTs should be used in this way. It is not intended that guidelines commended for health authorities in this way should be used as instructions to patients and clinicians at a local level. Other UK organizations appraising the validity of existing guidelines include the National Institute for Clinical Excellence (NICE) and the Scottish Intercollegiate Guidelines Network (SIGN). In the USA, the NGC has explicit inclusion criteria for adopting guidelines and an extensive checklist used to summarize and evaluate individual guidelines.

Second, guidelines may be appraised at the clinical level. How can an individual form a judgement as to whether a guideline is well constructed and likely to be useful? Various methods have been suggested (e.g. Palmer, 1999; Warner and Blizard, 1998; see Table) for the critical appraisal of guidelines. Such an approach examines the validity of the guideline, its content and its applicability to the clinical situation in hand. A critical approach to guidelines may be particularly useful when there are multiple sets of guidelines relating to a particular issue, e.g. the drug treatment of Alzheimer's disease (Harvey, 1999) or the management of depression in general practice (Littlejohns *et al*, 1999).

Finally, the quality of guidelines can be empirically examined against established methodological standards. Shaneyfelt *et al* (1999) found that published guidelines did not adhere well to methodological standards, especially in

Critical appraisal of clinical guidelines

Are the recommendations valid?
Is the target population specified?
Who are the intended users?
Does the guideline specify who developed it and is the methodology of its construction available?
Are any potential conflicts of interest declared?
Were all options and outcomes considered?
Was an explicit and sensible process used to identify, select and combine evidence?
Was an explicit and sensible process used to consider the relative value of different outcomes?
Is the guideline likely to account for important recent developments?
Has a cost analysis been performed?
Has the guideline been subjected to peer review and testing?
How recent is the guideline and does it have an expiry date?

What are the recommendations?
Are practical clinically important recommendations made?
How strong are the recommendations?

Are there subgroups within the target population who are particularly likely to benefit?
Any subgroups who will not benefit, or may even be harmed?
What is the impact of uncertainty associated with the evidence and values used in the guidelines?

Will the recommendations help me in caring for my patient?
Is the primary objective of the guidelines consistent with my objective?
Are the recommendations applicable to my patient?
Is my patient likely to benefit from following the guideline's recommendations?
Is my patient likely to suffer any potential risks or adverse consequences?
Are the resources available to implement the recommendations?

After Warner JP, Blizzard R (1998) How to appraise clinical guidelines. Psychiatric Bulletin **22**: 759–61.

the area of identification and summary of the evidence. There was only a modest improvement with more recently published guidelines. Grilli *et al* (2000) were critical of practice guidelines developed by speciality societies, on the grounds that most of them did not involve other stakeholders, such as public agencies or patient groups.

Using clinical guidelines

It appears that most clinicians are favourably disposed towards clinical guidelines (Renvoize *et al*, 1997). However, most clinicians and service providers will not wish to produce their own guidelines from scratch. There is no need for them to do so, since there may already be existing guidance. Besides, the resources required to produce a new set of guidelines may be excessive for a small organization like a primary care trust or an old age psychiatry service. It is more likely the clinicians will adopt or modify published guidance, preferably after suitable appraisal as suggested above.

Guidelines may be used as a source of advice on the management of a condition or the use of an intervention (Feder *et al*, 1999). They usually have a broader scope than systematic reviews, which tend to focus on an individual problem or intervention. They can provide a coherent and integrated view on how to manage a condition.

Guidelines can also have an important role in continuing medical education, as a source of information, for self assessment or to identify gaps in knowledge and performance, particularly where measurable criteria are provided with the guidelines. Clinicians may also use guidelines as part of an evidence-based approach to solving clinical questions (Feder *et al*, 1999).

Following the choice of which guideline to adopt, the separate stages of dissemination, implementation and monitoring all require attention if a guideline is to be successful in the aim of helping clinicians to provide better and more consistent care to their patients (Forrest *et al*, 1996).

Developing a guideline is, of course, no guarantee that it will be taken up by clinicians and, even then, there is no certainty that it will lead to demonstrable improvements in patient care. It has frequently been noted how difficult it is to change the practice of clinicians even when there is good evidence for them do so. Evaluating the impact and the effectiveness of guidelines is a potentially complex and expensive business. Resources and motivation to perform the appropriate evaluations are often lacking (Andrews, 1999).

Spreading the word . . .

Several key issues in the dissemination of guidelines have been identified (Thomson *et al*, 1995). These include being clear as to the intended target users of the guideline and considering how and by what means this group can be reached. The form in which the guideline is to be presented

must be considered. Possible methods might include, for example, induction material for junior doctors, on posters, as a separate document, in a journal, electronically, in patient literature, or in any combination of these. It may be necessary to customize the means by which the information is presented to achieve maximum impact (Langley *et al*, 1998). Guidelines may be presented in partial form by way of prompts and reminders, for example the use of a distinctive logo. Whether to establish regular dissemination, for example six monthly to new trainee doctors, also needs to be decided.

Evaluation needs to consider various issues (Thomson *et al*, 1995). These include ascertaining whether the guidelines have been received, read, used and locally endorsed or evaluated. Several methods are available to assess guideline uptake, including surveys, questionnaires, case note reviews and routine monitoring. Who will be responsible for evaluation and with what resources? How will changes be incorporated, by whom and how often? Perhaps guidelines should only be issued with an expiry date on them.

Why guidelines are sometimes not taken up and what factors can improve their incorporation into practice are important questions (Davis and Taylor-Vaisey, 1997). For example, ensuring that the guidelines reach the target audience is crucial. Accompanying dissemination with educational interventions is effective (Thomas *et al*, 1999), as is promotion and endorsement by peers (especially local clinical leaders), whereas publication in journals seems to be ineffective. Both organizational support (Curry, 2000; Solberg, 2000) and information technology support (Lobach and Hammond, 1997; Owens, 1998) are also required. Corb *et al* (1999) examined the components of information systems that should promote effective guideline implementation.

Overall, it appears that a single strategy aimed at the individual clinician is unlikely to be effective. Instead, implementation strategies should incorporate several approaches, taking into account the nature of the guideline and the organization where it is being disseminated (Moulding *et al*, 1999; Ockene and Zapke, 2000; Solberg *et al*, 2000). However, not all multifaceted interventions are effective (Wensing *et al*, 1998), so further work is clearly needed.

Are guidelines effective?

Do guidelines change the behaviour of clinicians and, if so, does this improve patient outcomes? Unless this happens, the expense and effort in producing and promoting the guidelines are of little value.

Advocates of guidelines have often been surprised to find that disseminating reviews and recommendations is insufficient to change clinical practice (Woolf and George, 2000). This has sometimes led to disillusionment (Aust and Ohman, 2000), though in other cases at least some changes in practice have been documented (Thomas *et al*, 2000).

There are several potential barriers to guideline adherence, including awareness, familiarity, lack of agreement and inertia (Cabana *et al*, 1999). Physician self-reporting of guideline adherence may be unreliable (Adams *et al*, 1999), so other methods of assessing adherence should be used as well. Those methods that effectively promote the uptake of guidelines are also likely to be successful in improving adherence to them in clinical practice (Woolf and George, 2000).

There is relatively little research on the crucial question of guidelines and clinical outcomes. Dowie (1998) reported on a number of studies in progress in general practice across the UK to evaluate clinical guidelines, including in some cases economic evaluations of the intervention packages. A systematic review (Worrall *et al*, 1997) found little evidence that guidelines had improved patient outcomes in primary care, but acknowledged that many studies used older guidelines and methods that may have been insensitive to small differences in outcomes. Doubtless this issue will be the focus of much research over the next few years (Jankowski 2001).

Possible shortcomings of guidelines

Guidelines may be slow and expensive to produce, especially if they are to be based on a systematic review of the literature. They are often of variable quality and they may be harmful to patients if they do not advocate the best options for patients (Woolf, 1998). Updating them may prove difficult as the resources that developed them initially may no longer be available. The most serious problem is that they may simply not be used in practice (Godlee, 1998). There are currently no agreed rules for how to manage rivalries between guidelines which cover the same clinical area.

It may be superficially attractive to include guidelines into health commissioning, as a means by which health commissioning authorities can influence clinicians, but in reality this may be counterproductive unless there is a sense of local ownership of the guidance. Organizations require time in order to assimilate guidelines and, if necessary, to modify them to their own local needs. In the end, the real 'consumers' of guidelines are clinicians and their patients (Saltman, 1998), so it is the utility of the guidelines for consumers which is at issue.

It is also important to realize that guidelines are not designed to, nor can they be expected to, anticipate all situations. In resistant depression, for example, it would be very difficult to develop evidence-based guidelines beyond one or two antidepressants as it would be impossible to perform adequate RCTs. In reality, only a small part of clinical practice is likely to be standardized by central direction. Following guidelines may be a useful indicator of quality, but it must be recognized that more complex cases may require other approaches, especially from specialist services. Clinical practice will always require clinical judgement in the individual case (Fletcher, 1998) and

clinicians also need to consider the needs and wishes of the individual patient. Furthermore, specialist clinicians probably have a responsibility to be 'ahead' of the officially sanctioned guidelines, in order to incorporate innovation and also to identify potential areas for new guidelines to be developed (Kennedy, 1999).

Another difficulty is that the situation in clinical practice may be more complex than the guidelines allow for. For example, to consider depression in primary care, the diagnosis may be more difficult to make, particularly with less severe degrees of depression, general practitioners may be reluctant to prescribe for what appear to be social problems, and patients themselves may be reluctant to take medication. All these factors may mitigate against the success of clinical guidelines in producing better outcomes (Kendrick, 2000). It is also suggested that many general practitioners may not even share the evidence-based medicine paradigm (Tomlin *et al*, 1999).

For the clinician, guidelines may induce a sense of wariness. For whose benefit are they being developed? The establishment of guidelines for a particular condition is one way in which a professional group may seek to increase its influence. Guidelines thus could be seen as carrying a mark of tribalism or being a source of power. Do guidelines hold you to account or is the mark of the expert having the authority to diverge from guidance in difficult cases? Or are guidelines a way of controlling maverick clinicians on the fringes of practice? Conversely, they may be a means of preserving clinical autonomy from managers and insurers by providing demonstrable evidence of clinical quality.

Legal issues

A final question concerns legal liability. There are two aspects to this: the responsibility of those introducing the guidelines and the liability for deviating from practice as laid down in a guideline (NHS Executive, 1996). The authors of guidelines presumably have responsibility for the quality of the information used, but not for the effects in clinical cases. Where guidelines are made mandatory, then the authority applying those restrictions to the decision-making ability of others is responsible. This is another reason why it is unsound for commissioning authorities to impose guidelines as mandatory in health agreements.

In the UK, the use of clinical guidelines is yet to produce large numbers of negligence cases. Under the 'Bolam test' (after the case of that name), there is already a defence that there may be two or more schools of thought on any particular aspect of clinical care. Besides, it could often be argued that the circumstances in the individual case may lie outside the applicability of the guideline. Nonetheless, deviation from a universally supported and adopted guideline would require good justification. Such a deviation would be best supported by having good and clear reasons, by demonstrating adequate consultation and by clear documentation in the medical notes. Similarly, in the Netherlands (Buijsen, 2000), judges increasingly refer to clinical guidelines, but they are not regarded as legal rules and, in general, clinical autonomy has been upheld.

References

Adams AS, Soumerai SB, Lomas J, Ross-Degnan D (1999) Evidence of self-report bias in assessing adherence to guidelines. *International Journal of Quality Health Care* 11: 187–92.

Andrews G (1999) Randomised controlled trials in psychiatry: important but poorly accepted. *British Medical Journal* 319: 562–4.

Aust B, Ohmann C (2000) Previous experiences with the evaluation of guidelines: disillusionment after an enthusiastic start. *Z Arztl Fortbild Qualitatssich* 94: 365–71.

Banerjee S, Dickinson E (1997) Evidence based health care in old age psychiatry. *International Journal of Psychiatry in Medicine* 27: 283–92.

Buijsen MA (2000) The legal significance of clinical guidelines in the Netherlands. *Medicine and Law* 19: 181–8.

Cabana MD, Rand CS, Powe NR, Wu AW, Wilson MH, Abboud PA, Rubin HR (1999) Why don't physicians follow clinical practice guidelines? A framework for improvement. *Journal of the American Medical Association* 282: 1458–65.

Cluzeau F, Littlejohns P, Grimshaw J, Feder G (1997) *Appraisal Instrument for Clinical Guidelines.* London: St George's Hospital Medical School.

Cook DJ, Greengold NL, Ellrodt AG, Weingarten SR (1997) The relation between systematic reviews and practice guidelines. *Annals of International Medicine* 127: 210–16.

Corb GJ, Liaw Y, Brandt CA, Shiffman RN (1999) An object-oriented framework for the development of computer-based guideline implementations. *Methods of Information in Medicine* 38: 148–53.

Curry SJ (2000) Organizational interventions to encourage guideline implementation. *Chest* 118: 40S–46S.

Davis DA, Taylor-Vaisey A (1997) Translating guidelines into practice: a systemic review of theoretic concepts, practical experience and research evidence in the adoption of clinical practice guidelines. *Canadian Medical Association Journal* 157: 408–16.

Dowie R (1998) A review of research in the United Kingdom to evaluate the implementation of clinical guidelines in general practice. *Family Practice* 15: 462–70.

Feder G, Eccles M, Grol R, Griffiths C, Grimshaw J (1999) Using clinical guidelines. *British Medical Journal* 318: 728–30.

Fletcher RH (1998) Practice guidelines and the practice of medicine: is it the end of clinical judgement and expertise? *Schweizerische Medizinische Wochenschrift* 28: 1883–8.

Forrest D, Hoskins A, Hussey R (1996) Clinical guidelines and their implementation. *Postgraduate Medical Journal* 72: 19–22.

Godlee F (1998) Getting evidence into practice. *British Medical Journal* 317: 6.

Greenwood R (1999) Clinical guidelines, clinical effectiveness and clinical governance. In: *A Practical Guide to Developing and Using Clinical Guidelines to Improve Clinical Practice.* London: Healthcare Events.

Grilli R, Magrini N, Penna A, Mura G, Liberati A (2000) Practice guidelines developed by specialty societies: the need for a critical appraisal. *Lancet* 355: 103–6.

Harvey R (1999) A review and commentary on a sample of 15 UK guidelines for the drug treatment of Alzheimer's disease. *International Journal of Geriatric Psychiatry* 14: 249–56.

Jankowski R (2001) Implementing national guidelines at local level. *BMJ* 322: 1258–9.

Kendrick T (2000) Why can't GPs follow guidelines on depression? *British Medical Journal* 320: 200–1.

Kennedy P (1999) Clinical governance in mental health services. 1. A chief executive's perspective. *Psychiatric Bulletin* 23: 711–14.

Langley C, Faulkner A, Watkins C, Gray S, Harvey I (1998) Use of guidelines in primary care – practitioners' perspectives. *Family Practice* 15: 105–11.

Littlejohns P, Cluzeau F, Bale R, Grimshaw G, Feder G, Moran S (1999) The quantity and quality of clinical practice guidelines for the management of depression in primary care in the UK. *British Journal of General Practice* 49: 205–10.

Lobach DF, Hammond WE (1997) Computerized decision support based on a clinical practice guideline improves compliance with care standards. *American Journal of Medicine* 102: 89–98.

Maisonneuve H, Cordier H, Durocher A, Matillon Y (1997) The French clinical guidelines and medical references programme: development of 48 guidelines for private practice over a period of 18 months. *J Eval Clin Pract* 3: 3–13.

Moulding NT, Silagy CA, Weller DP (1999) A framework for effective management of change in clinical practice: dissemination and implementation of clinical practice guidelines. *Quality in Health Care* 8: 177–83.

NHS Executive (1996) *Clinical Guidelines: Using Clinical Guidelines to Improve Patient Care in the NHS.* London: Department of Health.

Ockene JK, Zapka JG (2000) Provider education to promote implementation of clinical practice guidelines. *Chest* 118: 33S–39S.

Owens DK (1998) Use of medical informatics to implement and develop clinical practice guidelines. *Western Journal of Medicine* 168: 166–75.

Palmer C (1999) *Evidence-base Briefing: Dementia.* London: Gaskell.

Renvoize EB, Hampshaw SM, Pinder JM, Ayres P (1997) What are hospitals doing about clinical guidelines? *Quality in Health Care* 6: 187–91.

Saltman DC (1998) Guidelines for every person. *Journal of Evaluation in Clinical Practice* **4**: 1–9.

Shaneyfelt TM, Mayo-Smith MF, Rothwangl J (1999) Are guidelines following guidelines? The methodological quality of clinical practice guidelines in the peer-reviewed medical literature. *Journal of the American Medical Association* **281**: 1900–5.

Solberg LI (2000) Guideline implementation: what the literature doesn't tell us. *Joint Commission Journal on Quality Improvement* **26**: 525–37.

Solberg LI, Brekke ML, Fazio CJ, Fowles J, Jacobsen DN, Kottke TE, Mosser G, O'Connor PJ, Ohnsorg KA, Rolnick SJ (2000) Lessons from experienced guideline implementers: attend to many factors and use multiple strategies. *Joint Commission Journal on Quality Improvement* **26**: 171–88.

Thomas L, Cullum N, McColl E, Rousseau N, Soutter J, Steen N (2000) Guidelines in professions allied to medicine. *Cochrane Database Syst Rev* CD000349.

Thomas LH, McColl E, Cullum N, Rousseau N, Soutter J (1999) Clinical guidelines in nursing, midwifery and the therapies: a systematic review. *Journal of Advanced Nursing* **30**: 40–50.

Thomson R, Lavender M, Madhok R (1995) How to ensure that guidelines are effective. *British Medical Journal* **311**: 237–42.

Tomlin Z, Humphrey C, Rogers S (1999) General practitioners' perceptions of effective health care. *British Medical Journal* **318**: 1532–5.

Trickey H, Harvey I, Wilcock G, Sharp D (1998) Formal consensus and consultation: a qualitative method for development of a guideline for dementia. *Quality in Health Care* **7**: 192–9.

Warner JP, Blizard R (1998) How to appraise clinical guidelines. *Psychiatric Bulletin* **22**: 759–61.

Wensing M, van der Weijden T, Grol R (1998) Implementing guidelines and innovations in general practice: which interventions are effective? *British Journal of General Practice* **48**: 991–7.

Woolf SH (1998) Do clinical guidelines define good medical care? The need for good science and the disclosure of uncertainty when defining 'best practices'. *Chest* **113**: 166S–171S.

Woolf SH, George JN (2000) Evidence-based medicine: interpreting studies and setting policy. *Hematology/Oncology Clinics of North America* **14**: 761–4.

Worrall G, Chaulk P, Freake D (1997) The effects of clinical practice guidelines on patient outcomes in primary care: a systematic review. *Canadian Medical Association Journal* **156**: 1705–12.

The authors receive occasional honoraria and hospitality from companies involved in the manufacture and marketing of drugs for older people.

Note

TRD is a part-time Senior Professional Adviser to the Department of Health in London. However, the content of this book and any views expressed are entirely those of the authors.

Chapter 1

Dementia

International Classification of Diseases (ICD 10)

Reference   WHO (1992) *International Classification of Diseases*, 10th edn. World Health Organization

Purpose

To describe clinical criteria for dementia and Alzheimer's disease.

Dementia is a syndrome due to disease of the brain, usually of a chronic or progressive nature, in which there is impairment of multiple higher cortical functions, including memory, thinking, orientation, comprehension, calculation, learning capacity, language and judgement. Consciousness is not clouded. The cognitive impairments are commonly accompanied, and occasionally preceded, by deterioration in emotional control, social behaviour, or motivation. This syndrome occurs in Alzheimer's disease, in cerebrovascular disease, and in other conditions primarily or secondarily affecting the brain.

In assessing the presence or absence of a dementia, special care should be taken to avoid false-positive identification; motivational or emotional factors, particularly depression, in addition to motor slowness and general physical frailty, may account for failure to perform, rather than loss of intellectual capacity.

Dementia produces a definite decline in intellectual functioning, and usually also some interference with personal activities of daily living, such as washing, dressing, eating, personal hygiene, excretory and toilet activities. How such a decline shows itself will depend a great deal on the social and cultural setting in which the subject lives. Changes in role performance, such as a decline in the ability to keep or find a job, should not be used as criteria of dementia because of the large cross-cultural differences that exist in what is appropriate, and the frequent occurrence of externally imposed changes upon the availability of work even within cultures.

If depressive symptoms are present but the criteria of depressive episode are not fulfilled, their presence can be recorded by means of a fifth digit, and similarly for hallucinations and delusions:

.×0   without additional symptoms.
.×1   other symptoms, predominantly delusional
.×2   other symptoms, predominantly hallucinatory
.×3   other symptoms, predominantly depressive
.×4   other mixed symptoms

Diagnostic Guidelines

. . . the primary requirement is evidence of a decline in both memory and thinking which is of a degree sufficient to impair personal activities of daily living. The impairment of memory is typically in the registration, storage and retrieval of new information previously learned and familiar material may also be lost particularly in the later stages. Dementia is more than dysmnesia, there is also impairment of thinking, the capacity for reasoning and a reduction of the flow of ideas. Processing of incoming information is impaired and the individual finds it increasingly difficult to attend to more than one stimulus at a time, such as taking part in a conversation with several persons and there is difficulty in shifting the focus of attention from one topic to another. If dementia is the sole diagnosis then evidence of a clear consciousness is required. However, a double diagnosis of delirium superimposed on dementia is common. The above symptoms and impairments should have been in evidence for at least 6 months for a confident clinical diagnosis of dementia to be made.

Dementia in Alzheimer's disease – ICD10 (reproduced with permission from ICD10, World Health Organization, Geneva)

Alzheimer's disease is a primary degenerative cerebral disease of unknown aetiology with characteristic neuropathological and neurochemical features. It is usually insidious in onset and slowly but steadily develops over a period of several years. This can be as short as two or three years, but can occasionally be considerably longer. The onset can be in middle adult life or even earlier (Alzheimer's disease of presenile onset), but the incidence is higher in later life (Alzheimer's disease of senile onset). In cases with onset before the age of 65–70, there is a trend towards their having a family history of a similar dementia, a more rapid course, and prominence of features of temporal and parietal lobe damage, including dysphasia or dyspraxia. In cases with a later onset, the course tends to be slower and to be characterized by a more general impairment of the higher cortical functions. Patients with Down's syndrome have a high risk of developing Alzheimer's disease.

There are characteristic changes in the brain: a marked reduction in the population of neurons, particularly in the hippocampus, substantia innominata, locus coeruleus; the temporo-parietal and frontal cortex; appearance of neurofibrillary tangles made of paired helical filaments; neurotic (argentophil) plaques which consist largely of amyloid and show a definite progression in their development (but plaques without amyloid are also known to exist); and granulovacuolar bodies. Neurochemical changes have also been found. These include a marked reduction in the neurotransmitters and neuromodulators.

As originally described, the clinical features are accompanied by the above brain changes. However, it now appears that the two do not always progress in parallel: one may be indisputably present with only minimal evidence of the other. Nevertheless the clinical features of Alzheimer's disease are such that it is often possible to make a presumptive diagnosis on clinical grounds alone.

1. Presence of a dementia as described above
2. Insidious onset with slow deterioration. While the onset seems usually difficult to pinpoint in time, realization by others that the defects exist may come suddenly. The plateau may appear to occur in the progression. Dementia in Alzheimer's disease is at present irreversible
3. Absence of clinical evidence or findings from special investigations which suggest that the mental state may be due to other systemic or brain disease which can induce a dementia (e.g. hypothyroidism, hypercalcaemia, vitamin B_{12} deficiency, niacin deficiency, neurosyphilis, normal pressure hydrocephalus or subdural haematoma)
4. Absence of a sudden apoplectic onset or of neurological signs of focal damage such as hemiparesis, sensory loss, visual field defect and incoordination occurring early in the illness (but such phenomena may be superimposed later).

Diagnostic Criteria for Research (based on ICD 10)

Reference   WHO (1992) *International Classification of Diseases.* 10th edn. World Health Organization

Purpose
To describe research criteria for the dementia.

Diagnostic criteria for research – ICD10 (reproduced with permission from ICD10, World Health Organization, Geneva)

Dementia
A. Evidence of a dementia, of a specified level of severity, based on the presence of each of the following:
1. A decline in memory which is most evident in the learning of new information, and in more severe cases, the recall of previously learned information is also affected. The impairment applies to both verbal and non-verbal material. The decline should be objectively verifiable and not based on subjective complaint. This should be achieved by obtaining a history from an informant and/or by neuropsychological testing. The level of severity should be assessed as follows:
Mild impairment: a degree of memory loss sufficient to interfere with everyday activities, though not so severe as to be incompatible with independent living. The main function affected is the learning of new material, but in early or mild cases, the medium and long-term memory may be affected little or not at all. For example, the individual has difficulty in registering, storing and recalling elements in daily living, such as where belongings have been put, social arrangements, or information recently imparted by family members.
Moderate impairment: a more severe degree of memory loss. Only highly learned or very familiar material is retained. New information is retained only occasionally and very briefly. The individual is unable to recall basic information about where he lives, what he has recently been doing, or the names of familiar persons. This degree of memory impairment is a serious handicap to independent living. An associated finding may be the intermittent loss of sphincter control.
Severe impairment: severe memory loss with only fragments of previously learned information remaining, the subject fails to recognize even close relatives. There is no retention of new information. The individual is not able to function in the community without close supervision: there is gross decline in personal care and loss of sphincter control of the bladder.
2. A decline in intellectual abilities characterized by deterioration in thinking and in the processing of information. Evidence for this should be obtained when possible from interviewing an informant and from a neuropsychological examination (if an estimate of premorbid intelligence can be made). To obtain both is desirable. Deterioration from a previously higher level of performance should be established by demonstration that the current level of handling and comprehension of ideas is incompatible with what might have been expected before. The level of intellectual impairment should be assessed as follows:
Mild impairment: the decline in intellectual abilities causes impaired performance in daily living, but not to a degree making the individual dependent on others. More complicated daily tasks or recreational activities cannot be undertaken.
Moderate impairment: the decline in intellectual abilities makes the individual unable to function without the assistance of another in daily living, including shopping and handling money. Within the home, only simple chores are preserved. Interests are very restricted and poorly sustained.
Severe impairment: the decline precludes not only independence from the assistance of others, but is characterized by an absence, or virtual absence, of intelligible ideation.
The overall severity of the dementia is best expressed as the level of memory or intellectual impairment, whichever is the more severe (e.g. mild memory impairment and moderate intellectual impairment indicates a dementia of moderate severity).
B. Absence of clouding of consciousness during a period of time long enough to enable the unequivocal demonstration of A. There may nevertheless be superimposed episodes of delirium in the course of a dementing illness. If a case presents with delirium, the diagnosis of dementia should be deferred because the impairment of thinking, memory and other higher functioning could be wholly attributed to the delirium itself.
C. A deterioration in emotional control, social behaviour or motivation. The change in emotional control may manifest itself as a depressive change in character, as unconcern or unawareness or as increased irritability. Social behaviour may become coarsened, with disregard for dress or eating habits, or unaccustomed coarseness in speech. The change in motivation is usually characterized by inertia or apathy.
D. For a confident clinical diagnosis, A should have been clearly present for at least six months; if the period since the manifest onset is shorter, the diagnosis can only be tentative.

The diagnosis is further supported by evidence of damage to other higher cortical functions, such as aphasia, agnosia, apraxia; and of disintegration of social behaviour and a progressive change in personality, in which reduced spontaneity is a conspicuous early feature.

Where facilities allow, the clinical diagnosis of dementia, and particularly of Alzheimer's type and vascular dementias, can be greatly assisted by the use of brain imaging techniques (computerized axial tomography, positron emission tomography, or nuclear magnetic resonance). The electroencephalogram may also be valuable although a negative EEG does not exclude Alzheimer's disease.

The diagnosis is confirmed by neuropathological examination.

Dementia in Alzheimer's disease

A. *Evidence of a dementia of a specific level of severity as set out under the general description of dementia.*

B. *Absence of evidence from the history, physical examination or special investigations for a clinically diagnosable cause for the dementia (e.g. head injury, multi-infarct dementia, normal pressure hydrocephalus, subdural haematoma, hypothyroidism, vitamin B_{12} or folic acid deficiency, niacin deficiency, hypercalcaemia, neurosyphilis or alcohol or drug-induced), a primary or secondary brain disease such as Huntington's or Parkinson's disease.*

The following features support the diagnosis, but are not necessary elements:

1. *involvement of cortical functions as evidence by aphasia, agnosia or apraxia;*
2. *decrease of motivation and drive, leading to apathy and lack of spontaneity; irritability and disinhibition of social behaviour;*
3. *evidence from special investigations that there is cerebral atrophy, particularly if this can be shown to be increasing over time;*
4. *in advanced, severe cases, there may be Parkinson-like extrapyramidal changes, logoclonia, and epileptic fits.*

DSM-IIIR: Diagnostic and Statistical Manual of Mental Disorders, Third Edition, revised
DSM-IV: Diagnostic and Statistical Manual of Mental Disorders, Fourth Edition

References   American Psychiatric Association: Diagnostic and Statistical Manual of Mental Disorders, Third Edition, revised. Washington DC, American Psychiatric Association, 1987. American Psychiatric Association: Diagnostic and Statistical Manual of Mental Disorders, Fourth Edition. Washington DC, American Psychiatric Association, 1994

Purpose

To describe clinical criteria for the condition.

DSMIII-R criteria for diagnosis of dementia (reprinted with permission from the Diagnostic and Statistical Manual of Mental Disorders, Third Edition. Copyright 1987 American Psychiatric Association)

A. *Demonstrable evidence of impairment in short- and long-term memory. Impairment in short-term memory (inability to learn new information) may be indicated by inability to remember three objects after 5 minutes. Long-term memory impairment (inability to remember information that was known in the past) may be indicated by inability to remember past personal information (e.g. what happened yesterday, birthplace, occupation) or facts of common knowledge (e.g. past Presidents, well-known dates).*

B. *At least one of the following:*
   (i)   *Impairment in abstract thinking, as indicated by inability to find similarities and differences between related words, difficulty in defining words and concepts, and other similar tasks*
   (ii) *Impaired judgment, as indicated by inability to make reasonable plans to deal with interpersonal, family and job-related problems and issues*
   (iii) *Other disturbances of higher cortical function such as aphasia (disorder of language), apraxia (inability to carry out motor activities despite intact comprehension and motor function), agnosia (failure to recognize or identify objects despite intact sensory function) and 'constructional difficulty' (e.g. inability to copy three-dimensional figures, assemble blocks or arrange sticks in specific designs).*
   (iv) *Personality change, i.e. alteration or accentuation of premorbid traits.*

C. *The disturbance in A and B significantly interferes with work or usual social activities or relationships with others.*

D. *Not occurring exclusively during the course of delirium.*

E. *Either (i) or (ii):*
   (i) *There is evidence from the history, physical examination, or laboratory tests of a specific organic factor (or factors) judged to be aetiologically related to the disturbance*
   (ii) *In the absence of such evidence, an aetiologic organic factor can be presumed if the disturbance cannot be account for by any non-organic mental disorder, e.g. major depression accounting for cognitive impairment.*

Criteria for severity of dementia:

Mild: *although work or social activities are significantly impaired, the capacity for independent living remains, with adequate personal hygiene and relatively intact judgment*
Moderate: *independent living is hazardous and some degree of supervision is necessary*
Severe: *activities of daily living are so impaired that continual supervision is required, e.g. unable to maintain minimal personal hygiene; largely incoherent or mute.*

Diagnostic criteria for dementia of the Alzheimer's type

A The development of multiple cognitive deficits manifested by both
  (1) memory impairment (impaired ability to learn new information or to recall previously learned information)
  (2) one (or more) of the following cognitive disturbances:
    (a) aphasia (language disturbance)
    (b) apraxia (impaired ability to carry out motor activities despite intact motor function)
    (c) agnosia (failure to recognize or identify objects despite intact sensory function)
    (d) disturbance in executive functioning (i.e., planning, organizing, sequencing, abstracting)

B The cognitive deficits in Criteria A1 and A2 each cause significant impairment in social or occupational functioning and represent a significant decline from a previous level of functioning

C The course is characterized by gradual onset and continuing cognitive decline

D The cognitive deficits in Criteria A1 and A2 are not due to any of the following:
  (1) other central nervous system conditions that cause progressive deficits in memory and cognition (e.g., cerebrovascular disease, Parkinson's disease, Huntingdon's disease, subdural hematoma, normal-pressure hydrocephalus, brain tumor)
  (2) systemic conditions that are known to cause dementia (e.g., hypothyroidism, vitamin B_{12} of folic acid deficiency, niacin deficiency, hypercalcemia, neurosyphilis, HIV infection)
  (3) substance-induced conditions

E The deficits do not occur exclusively during the course of a delirium

F The disturbance is not better accounted for by another Axis 1 disorder (e.g., Major Depressive Disorder, Schizophrenia)

Code based on type of onset and predominant features
  With Early Onset: if onset is at age 65 years or below
    F00.01 With Delusions: if delusions are the predominant feature
    F00.03 With Depressed Mood: if depressed mood (including presentations that meet full symptom criteria for a Major Depressive Episode) is the predominant feature. A separate diagnosis for Mood Disorder Due to a General Medical Condition is not given.
    F00.00 Uncomplicated: if none of the above predominates in the current clinical presentation
  With Late Onset: if onset is after 65 years
    F00.11 With Delusions: if delusions are the predominant feature
    F00.13 With Depressed Mood: if depressed mood (including presentations that meet full symptom criteria for a Major Depressive Episode) is the predominant feature. A separate diagnosis of Mood Disorder Due to a General Medical Condition is not given.
    F00.10 Uncomplicated: if none of the above predominates in the current clinical presentation

Specify if
  With Behavioral Disturbance
  Coding note: Also code G30.0 Alzheimer's Disease, With Early Onset, or G30.1, Alzheimer's Disease, With Late Onset, on Axis III

Diagnostic criteria for F01.xx Vascular Dementia

A The development of multiple cognitive deficits manifested by both
  (1) memory impairment (impaired ability to learn new information or to recall previously learned information)
  (2) one (or more) of the following disturbances:
    (a) aphasia (language disturbance)
    (b) apraxia (impaired ability to carry out motor activities despite intact motor function)
    (c) agnosia (failure to recognize or identify objects despite intact sensory function)
    (d) disturbance in executive functioning (i.e., planning, organizing, sequencing, abstracting)

B The cognitive deficits in Criteria A1 and A2 each cause significant impairment in social or occupational functioning and represent a significant decline from a previous level of functioning.

C Focal neurological signs and symptoms (e.g., exaggeration of deep tendon reflexes, extensor plantar response, pseudobulbar palsy, gait abnormalities, weakness of an extremity) or laboratory evidence indicative of cerebrovascular disease (e.g., multiple infarctions involving cortex and underlying white matter) that are judged to be etiologically related to the disturbance.

D The deficits do not occur exclusively during the course of a delirium.

Code based on predominant features:
  F01.81 With Delusions: if delusions are the predominant feature
  F01.83 With Depressed Mood: if depressed mood (including presentations that meet full symptom criteria for a Major Depressive Episode) is the predominant feature. A separate diagnosis of Mood Disorder Due to a General Medical Condition is not given.
  F01.80 Uncomplicated: if none of the above predominates in the current clinical presentation.

Specify if
  With Behavioral Disturbance
  Coding note: also code cerebrovascular condition on Axis III.

Practice Parameter: Diagnosis of Dementia (an Evidence-Based Review)

Reference   Knopman DS, DeKosky ST, Cummings JL, Chui H, Corey-Bloom J, Relkin N, Small GW, Miller B and Stevens JC (2001). Practice parameter: diagnosis of dementia (an evidence-based review): report of the Quality Standards Subcommittee of the American Academy of Neurology. *Neurology* 56:1143–53

Summary

An update of the 1994 practice parameter for the diagnosis of dementia in the elderly

Four questions were addressed by examining published studies from 1985 to 1999 in English. The four questions were:

1. Are the current criteria for the diagnosis of dementia reliable?
2. Are the current diagnostic criteria able to establish a diagnosis for the prevalent dementias in the elderly?
3. Do laboratory tests improve the accuracy of the clinical diagnosis of dementing illness?
4. What comorbidities should be evaluated in elderly patients undergoing an initial assessment for dementia?

Practice recommendations

- DSM-IIIR definition of dementia, which is identical to the DSM-IV definition is reliable and should be used routinely (Guideline).
- The NINCDS-ADRDA for the diagnosis of probably Alzheimer's disease or DSM-IIIR criteria dementia of

Table 1 Classification of evidence

Class	Description
I	Evidence provided by a well designed prospective study in a broad spectrum of person with the suspected condition, using a ''gold standard'' for case definition, in which test is applied in a blinded evaluation, and enabling the assessment of appropriate tests of diagnostic accuracy.
II	Evidence provided by a well designed prospective study of a narrow spectrum of persons with the suspected condition, or a well designed retrospective study of a broad spectrum of persons with an established condition (by ''gold standard'') compared with a broad spectrum of controls, in which test is applied in blinded evaluation, and enabling the assessment of appropriate tests of diagnostic accuracy.
II	Evidence provided by a retrospective study in which either persons with the established condition or controls are of a narrow spectrum, and in which test is applied in a blinded evaluation.
IV	Any design in which test is not applied in blinded evaluation OR evidence provided by expert opinion alone or in descriptive case series (without controls).

Table 2

Recommendation	Description
Standard	Principle for patient management that reflects a high degree of clinical certainty (usually this requires Class I evidence that directly addresses the clinical question, or overwhelming Class II evidence when circumstances preclude randomized clinical trials).
Guideline	Recommendation for patient management that reflects moderate clinical certainty (usually this requires Class II evidence or a strong consensus of Class III evidence).
Practice Option	Strategy for patient management for which the clinical utility is uncertain (inconclusive or conflicting evidence or opinion).
Practice Advisory	Practice recommendation for emerging and/or newly approved therapies or technologies based on evidence from at least one Class I study. The evidence may demonstrate only a modest statistical effect or limited (partial) clinical response, or significant cost–benefit questions may exist. Substantial (or potential) disagreement among practitioners or between payers and practitioners may exist.

the Alzheimer type should be routinely used (Guideline)
- The Hatchinski Ischemic Index criteria may be of use in the diagnosis for cerebrovascular disease in dementia (Option)
- The Consortium for dementia with Lewy bodies diagnostic criteria may be of use in clinical practice (Option)
- The Consensus diagnostic criteria for fronto-temporal dementia may be of use in clinical practice (Option)
- Clinical criteria for Creutzfeldt-Jakob disease should be used in rapidly progressive dementia syndromes (Guideline)

The main conclusions were the criteria of probably Alzheimer's disease as good sensitivity for neuropathologic Alzheimer's disease but less optimal specificity. The clinical phenotypes embodied in the diagnostic criteria for vascular dementia, dementia with Lewy bodies, and fronto-temporal dementia do not map precisely onto neuropathologic phenotypes. Although there are strong clinical pathologic relationships for these disorders in the majority of patients, there are many patients with atypical or non-specific clinical presentations. The clinical phenotype of Creutzfeldt-Jakob disease is more tightly linked to its expected CJD pathology.

Do laboratory tests improve the accuracy of clinical diagnosis of dementing illness. (An immunoassay for the detection of the peptide in CSF with a specificity of 99% and sensitivity of 96% for the diagnosis of CJD (Hsich G, Kenney K & Gibbs C et al, 1996).

Conclusions

The CSF 14-3-3 protein assay is useful for confirming the diagnosis of CJD. In contrast, no laboratory tests have yet emerged that are appropriate for routine use in the clinical evaluation of patients with suspected Alzheimer's disease. Several promising avenues – genotyping, imaging and biomarkers – are being pursued, but proof that a laboratory test has value is arduous. Ultimately, the putative diagnostic test must be administered to a representative sample of patients with dementia who eventually have pathologic confirmation of their diagnoses. A valuable test will be one that increases diagnostic accuracy over and above a competent clinical diagnosis.

Practice recommendation

- Structural neuroimaging with either a non-contrast CT or MR scan in the routine initial evaluation of patients with dementia is appropriate (Guideline)
- Linear or volumetric MR or CT measurement strategies for the diagnosis of AD and are not recommended for routine use at this time (Guideline)
- For patients with suspected dementia, SPECT cannot be recommended for routine use in either initial or differential diagnosis as it has not demonstrated

superiority to clinical criteria (Guideline)
- PET imaging is not recommended for routine use in the diagnostic evaluation of dementia at this time (Guideline)
- Routine use or APOE genotyping in patients with suspected Alzheimer's disease is not recommended for routine use in the diagnosis of Alzheimer's disease
- There are no other genetic markers recommended for routine use in the diagnosis of Alzheimer's disease (Guideline)
- Testing for tau mutations of Alzheimer's disease gene mutations is not recommended for routine evaluation in patients with FTD at this time (Guideline)
- There are no CSF or other biomarkers recommended for routine use in determining the diagnosis of Alzheimer's disease at this time
- The CSF 14-3-3 protein is recommended for confirming or rejecting the diagnosis of CJD in clinically appropriate circumstances.

What comorbidities should be screened for in elderly patients undergoing an initial assessment for dementia?

Conclusions

Depression, B12 deficiency and hypothyroidism are comorbidities that are likely to appear in the elderly and in patients with suspected dementia in particular. Although treatment of these disorders may not completely reverse cognitive dysfunction, they should be recognized and treated. No new evidence has appeared since 1994 to support or refute the recommendation to perform "routine" blood tests in patients being evaluated for dementia.

Practice recommendations

- Depression is a common, treatable comorbidity in patients with dementia and should be screened for (Guideline)
- B12 deficiency is common in the elderly and B12 levels should be included in routine assessments of the elderly (Guideline)
- Because of its frequency, hypothyroidism should be screened for in elderly patients (Guideline)
- Unless the patient has some specific risk factor or evidence or prior syphilitic infection or resides in one of the few areas in the United States with high numbers of syphilis cases, screening for the disorder in patients with dementia is not justified (Guideline).

Reference

Hsich G, Kenney K & Gibbs C *et al* (1996). The 14-3-3 brain protein in cerebrospinal fluid is a marker for transmissible spongiform encephalopathies. *New England Journal of Medicine* 335:924–30

Practice Parameter: Early Detection of Dementia: Mild Cognitive Impairment (an Evidence-Based Review)

Reference   Peterson RC, Stevens JC, Ganguli M, Tangalos EG, Cummings JL, DeKosky ST (2001). Practice parameter: early detection of dementia: mild cognitive impairment (an evidence-based review): report of the Quality Standards Subcommittee of the American Academy of Neurology. *Neurology* 56: 1133–42

Purpose

The purpose of the reviews is to determine whether screening different groups of elderly individuals in a general or specialty practice would be beneficial in detecting dementia. The authors based their review on standardized, computerized literature searches. The classification of evidence was as follows:

Class I   Evidence provided by one or more well designed, randomized, controlled clinical trials, including overviews (meta-analyses) of such trials

Class II   Evidence provided by well designed observational studies with concurrent controls (e.g. case control or cohort studies)

Class III   Evidence provided by expert opinion, case series, case reports, and studies with historical controls

(47 references)

The levels of recommendation were:

Standard   Principle for patient management that reflects a high degree of clinical certainty. (Usually requires Class I evidence that directly addresses clinical questions or overwhelming Class II evidence when circumstances preclude randomized clinical trials)

Guideline   Recommendation for patient management that reflects moderate clinical certainty. (Usually requires Class II evidence or a strong consensus of Class III evidence)

Option   Strategy for patient management for which clinical utility is uncertain (inconclusive or conflicting evidence or opinion).

The conclusions from the primary question "Does the presence of mild cognitive impairment predict the development of dementia?" was that, taken together, the studies reviewed indicated that individuals characterized as being cognitively impaired but not meeting clinical criteria for dementia or Alzheimer's disease (mild cognitive impairment) have a high risk of progressing to dementia or Alzheimer's disease. If the figures for incident Alzheimer's disease from the general population are used, the rates range from 0.2% in the 65–69 age range to 3.9% in the 85–89 year range. The studies of mild cognitive impairment cited above indicated that the rate of progression to dementia or Alzheimer's disease is between 6% and 25% per year.

The recommendations were as follows:
Patients with mild cognitive impairment should be recognized and monitored for cognitive and functional decline due to their increased risk for subsequent dementia (guideline). General cognitive screening instruments e.g. Mini Mental State Examination should be considered for the detection of dementia in individuals with suspected cognitive impairment (guideline). Brief cognitive assessment instruments that focus on limited aspects of cognitive function (e.g. Clock Drawing Test, Time and Change Test) may be considered when screening patients for dementia (option). Neuropsychologic batteries should be considered useful in identifying patients with dementia, particularly when administered to a population at increased risk of cognitive impairment (guideline). Interview techniques may be considered in identifying patients with dementia, particularly in a population at increased risk of cognitive impairment (option).

Correspondence

Quality Standards Subcommittee
American Academy of Neurology
1080 Montreal Ave
St Paul
MN 55116
USA

Consortium to Establish a Registry for Alzheimer's Disease (CERAD)

References Morris JC, Heyman A, Mohs RC *et al.* (1989) CERAD Part I: Clinical and neuropsychological assessment of Alzheimer's disease. *Neurology* 39: 1159–65.

Mirra SS, Heyman A, McKeel DW *et al.* (1991) CERAD Part II: Standardization of the neuropathological assessment of Alzheimer's disease. *Neurology* 41: 479–86.

Mirra SS, Hart MN, Terry RD. (1993) Making the diagnosis of Alzheimer's disease: a primer for practicing pathologists. *Archives of Pathology and Laboratory Medicine* 117: 132–44.

Tariot PN, Mack JL, Patterson MB *et al.* (1995) The CERAD Behavior Rating Scale for Dementia. *American Journal of Psychiatry* 152: 1349–57.

Purpose

CERAD involved 24 Alzheimer's Disease Research Centers and University Medical Centers in the USA engaged in dementia research. The purpose of the consortium was to standardize procedures for the evaluation and diagnosis of patients with Alzheimer's disease.

Summary

CERAD has developed the following standardized instruments to assess the manifestation of Alzheimer's disease: clinical, neuropsychology, neuropathology, Behavior Rating Scale, and assessment of service needs.

Staff at participating clinical sites were initially trained and certified in the administration of the assessment instruments to screen carefully the subjects enrolled in the CERAD study. The Alzheimer's disease study population comprises 1094 patients and 463 non-demented elderly controls matched for age, sex and education. Cases and controls were evaluated at point of entry and annually thereafter, including (if possible) autopsy examination of the brain in order to track the natural progression of AD and to obtain neuropathological confirmation of clinical diagnosis. All of the data obtained with these instruments were pooled and maintained at the CERAD Methodology and Data Management Center at the University of Washington in Seattle. The CERAD database has become a major resource for research in Alzheimer's disease, containing up to 7 years of longitudinal data on the natural progression of the disorder and the correlation of clinical and neuropsychological manifestations and neuropathological changes.

There are three basic CERAD assessment packets, which consist of batteries of brief forms designed to gather demographic, clinical, neurological and neuropsychological data on demented subjects sufficient to establish a clinical diagnosis of dementia based on CERAD criteria.

The clinical battery consists of demographic data from the subject and informant, clinical history regarding cognitive function, systemic disorders, cerebrovascular disease, parkinsonism, depression, drug side effects, the Blessed Dementia Scale, behavioral abnormalities, Short Blessed Test, calculation, clock and language tests, physical examination (including neurological examination and screening for extrapyramidal dysfunction), laboratory and imaging studies, the Clinical Dementia Rating Scale and finally a diagnostic impression of either AD alone, AD associated with other disorders, or non-AD dementia.

The neuropsychological battery consists of the following tests: verbal fluency, a modified 15-item subset of the Boston Naming Test, Mini Mental State Examination, word list memory task recall and recognition, constructional praxis.

The CERAD neuropathology assessment is a highly respected instrument widely available in the USA and abroad for clinical and epidemiological studies of AD and other progressive dementias in the elderly. Its purpose was to establish more accurate, reliable and standardized neuropathological criteria for the diagnosis of AD and to develop a practical protocol for post-mortem examination of the brain which would provide standard, reliable measures for determining the neuropathological spectrum and heterogeneity of AD and other dementias. The assessment packet includes forms which gather information on demographic data, history, gross examination, cerebrovascular disease, microscopic vascular findings, major non-vascular microscopic findings, microscopic evaluation of hippocampus and neocortex, assessment of neurohistological findings and the final neuropathological diagnosis and assessment. It is accompanied by a detailed manual, *The CERAD Guide to Neuropathological Assessment of AD and Other Dementias.*

The Behavioral Rating Scale for Dementia (BRSD) is a standardized instrument for rating behavior abnormality in demented or cognitively impaired individuals. Items are scaled according to frequency of psychopathology. The scale is informant based and consists of 46 items which can be mapped onto six clinically relevant domains, such as depressive features, psychotic symptoms, behavioral dysregulation, irritability/agitation, vegetative features, aggression and affective lability. There is also a shorter 17-item version.

Assessment of service needs is a questionnaire that CERAD has developed for administration to caregivers of subjects with AD and that assesses the need and extent of use of the most common services needed for care of persons with dementia.

The questionnaire includes questions on the caregiver's current situation, overnight care for the patient outside the home, day care for the patient outside the home, care of the patient in the home, and other services.

Address for correspondence

Albert Heyman MD
Box 3203
University Medical Center
Durham, NC 27710, USA
stric007@mc.duke.edu

Recognition and Initial Assessment of Alzheimer's Disease and Related Dementias
Early Identification of Alzheimer's Disease and Related Dementias: Quick Reference Guide for Clinicians

Reference   Costa PT Jr, Williams TF, Somerfield M *et al* (1996) *Agency for Health Care Policy and Research (AHCPR) Clinical Practice No. 19.* Publications No. 97-0702/97-0703

Purpose

To increase the likelihood of early recognition and assessment of a potential dementing illness, so that concern can be eliminated, treatable conditions can be identified and addressed, and non-reversible conditions can be diagnosed early enough to permit the patient and family to plan for contingencies such as long-term care. The guidelines were developed using a private sector interdisciplinary panel comprising psychologists, psychiatrists, neurologists, interns, geriatricians, nurses, social workers and control representatives. The panel conducted extensive literature searches to identify empirical studies of assessment and mental status instruments. Results of literature reviews and meta-analysis were used to develop a draft guideline, which was further refined by subsequent peer review.

Purpose

The *Quick Reference Guide for Clinicians* was developed by a multidisciplinary panel of health care professionals and consumer representatives focusing on (1) symptoms that suggest the presence of dementia, and (2) steps to follow in conducting an initial assessment for Alzheimer's disease or a related dementia. Information is also provided about how to interpret test results, the role of neuropsychological testing and resources for patients and families facing a diagnosis of probable dementia.

Summary

(1) Symptoms that may indicate dementia

Does the person have increased difficulty with any of the activities listed below?

- *Learning and retaining new information.* Patient is more repetitive; has trouble remembering recent conversations, events, appointments; frequently misplaced objects
- *Handling complex tasks.* Patient has trouble following a complex train of thought or performing tasks that require many steps such as balancing a checkbook or cooking a meal
- *Reasoning ability.* Patient is unable to respond with a reasonable plan to problems as work or home, such as

knowing what to do if the bathroom is flooded; shows uncharacteristic disregard for rules of social conduct
- *Spatial ability and orientation.* Patient has trouble driving, organizing objects around the house, finding his or her way around familiar places
- *Language.* Patient has increasing difficulty with finding the words to express what he or she wants to say, and with following conversations.
- *Behavior.* Patient appears more passive and less responsive; is more irritable than usual; is more suspicious than usual; misinterprets visual or auditory stimuli.

In addition to noting failure to arrive at the right time for appointments, the clinician can look for difficulty discussing current events in an area of interest, and changes in behaviour or dress. It may also be helpful to follow up on areas of concern by asking the patient or family members relevant questions.

(2) Conducting an initial assessment

See flow chart.

Summary

The panel's major findings include:

1. Certain triggers should prompt the clinician to undertake an initial assessment for dementia.
2. An initial assessment should combine information from a focused history and physical examination and evaluation of mental and functional status, and from reliable informant reports. It should also include an assessment for delirium and depression.
3. An assessment instrument known as the Functional Activities Questionnaire is a particularly useful informant-based measure in the initial assessment of functional impairment in dementia.
4. Among various mental status tests, the Mini Mental State Examination, the Blessed Information Memory Concentration Test, the Blessed Orientation Memory Concentration Test and the Short Test of Mental Status are largely equivalent in terms of discriminative ability for early-stage dementia. Clinicians should assess and consider factors such as sensory impairment and physical

Early identification of Alzheimer's disease and related dementias

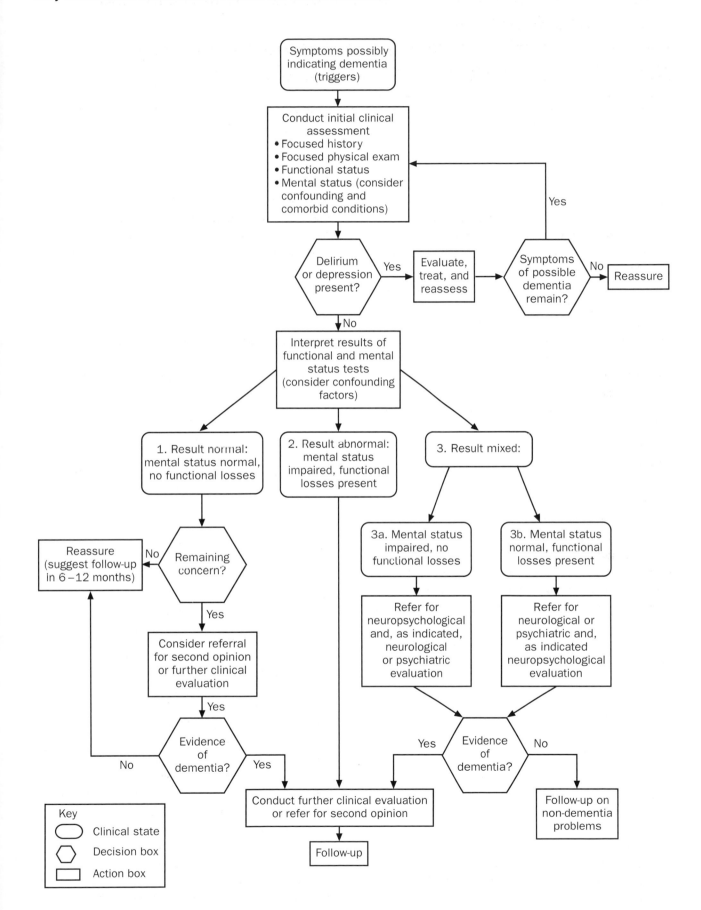

disability when selecting mental and functional status tests, and also social factors such as age, educational level and cultural influences in the interpretation of test results.

(See flowchart for recognition and initial assessment of Alzheimer's and related dementias.)

Assessment

A diagnosis of dementia requires a decline from the previous level of function, and impairment in multiple cognitive domains. Because evidence of decline from previous ability is critical in establishing dementia, personal knowledge of the patient is invaluable to the clinician. The focused history is critical. It is particularly important to establish the symptoms, mode of onset, progression and duration. A focused physical examination is an essential component of the initial assessment. Special emphasis should be placed on assessment for the conditions that cause delirium. A brief mental status test can be used, but is not diagnostic.

Assessment for depression

Depression can be difficult to distinguish from dementia. The clinical interview is the mainstay for evaluating and diagnosing depression in older adults. The Geriatric Depression Scale (GDS) and the Centre for Epidemiological Studies – Depression Scale (CES–D) are two depression-screening instruments that may be helpful.

Interpreting the findings

Three possible results can be obtained from the combination of findings of assessment and mental and functional status; normal, abnormal or mixed.

When the results of both mental and functional status tests are normal and there are no other clinical concerns, reassurance and suggested reassessment in 12 months is appropriate. If concerns persist, referral for a second opinion or further clinical evaluation should be considered.

When both mental and functional status tests reveal findings of abnormality, further clinical evaluation should be conducted. Laboratory tests should be conducted only after it has been confirmed that the patient has impairment in multiple domains that represents a decline from the previous level of functioning; if delirium and depression have been excluded; if family factors such as educational levels have been considered; and if medical conditions have been ruled out.

If there are mixed results – abnormal findings on the mental status tests with no abnormalities in functional status or *vice versa*, further evaluation is called for and may point to neurological, psychiatric or psychological problems.

The role of neuropsychological testing

Neuropsychological testing may be helpful in identifying dementia among persons with high pre-morbid intellectual functioning, in discriminating between patients with a dementing illness and those with focal cerebral disease, and in differentiating between certain causes of dementia.

Difficulties with the following might indicate a need for further assessment for the presence of dementia: learning and retaining new information; handling complex tasks; reasoning ability; spatial ability and orientation; language and behaviour.

Address for correspondence

AHCPR Clearing House
PO Box 8547
Silverspring, MD 20907-8547
USA

Early Diagnosis of Dementia: Which tests are indicated? What are their costs?

Reference Van Crevel H, van Gool WA, Walstra GJM (1999) Early diagnosis of dementia: which tests are indicated? What are their costs? *Journal of Neurology* 246: 73–8

Purpose

To describe a set of investigations that should be carried out in the setting of a memory clinic.

Summary

Dementia is reversible only in a minority of situations and the decision about which investigations to carry out has been the subject of much debate. Clinicians still regard it as an unforgivable sin to miss a treatable cause of anything, while on the other hand it is undesirable to subject people to unnecessary tests and procedures. The arguments for and against any particular type of investigation are considered in relation to three issues:

1. Reversible dementia is rare (about 1% of patients).
2. If the clinical criteria for diagnosing primary degenerative dementia are used consistently, the results of investigations can be predicted with sufficient accuracy, except those of blood tests.
3. Treatment of reversible dementia has the best results for the most frequent causes of the syndrome – depression and drug intoxication – however, some medical and surgical causes of dementia can also be effectively treated.

Recommendations

The guidelines propose the following diagnostic tests in the setting of the outpatient memory clinic.

1. *Blood tests*
   - diagnostic targets: (a) medical causes of reversible dementia (test below indicated with an asterisk); (b) secondary pathology, for example anaemia, diabetes, nutritional deficiency (tests below without an asterisk)
   - clinical prediction: insufficiently accurate; therefore:
   - as routine: thyroid function*, vitamin B_{12}*, syphilis, serology*, calcium*, renal* and liver* function, glucose, haemoglobin, haematocrit, vitamin B_{12} and folate.
2. *EEG*
   - diagnostic targets: (a) epilepsy, metabolic encephalopathies, Creutzfeldt-Jakob disease;

(b) differentiation between depression with severe cognitive impairment and AD with depression
   - clinical prediction: sufficiently accurate, therefore
   - on clinical indication (see 'diagnostic targets').
3. *CT or MRI scans*
   - diagnostic targets: (a) surgical causes of reversible dementia; (b) vascular causes of dementia
   - clinical prediction: sufficiently accurate; therefore:
   - on clinical indication (see 'diagnostic targets'). (Note: CT is sensitive enough for surgical causes of reversible dementia, but MRI may be preferable in some patients suspected of vascular dementia.)
4. *Other diagnostic tests*
   - on clinical indication, depending on the individual patient and specific diagnostic hypotheses, for example, if CNS infection is considered: examination of the cerebrospinal fluid.

The recommendation to perform diagnostic investigations other than blood tests in elderly demented patients, as clinically indicated, puts additional emphasis on the clinical evaluation. History (including that from an informant) and examination (including mental status) can never be replaced by ordering tests. The guidelines and their background make the clinician ask himself: does this patient have a history or signs of depression or drug intoxication? Are there clinical pointers to a surgical cause (normal pressure hydrocephalus, subdural haematoma, cerebral brain tumour)? Is a vascular cause possible? Or does this patient meet the criteria for primary degenerative dementia (mentioned above)? If yes, is there treatable secondary pathology?

Address for correspondence

H van Crevel
Dept of Neurology
Academic Medical Center
University of Amsterdam
PO Box 22700
1100 DE Amsterdam
The Netherlands

Guidelines for the Evaluation of Dementia and Age-related Cognitive Decline

Reference   The American Psychological Association (1998) *American Psychologist* 53: 1298–303

Purpose

Guidelines for clinical psychologists.

Summary

They are divided into:
General guideline (familiarity with nomenclature and diagnostic criteria).

1. Psychologists performing evaluations of dementia and age-related cognitive decline should be familiar with the prevailing diagnostic nomenclature and specific diagnostic criteria

General guidelines (ethical considerations)
2. Psychologists must attempt to obtain informed consent
3. Psychologists must gain specialized competence
4. Psychologists must seek and provide appropriate consultation
5. Psychologists must be aware of personal and societal biases and engage in nondiscriminatory practice

Procedural guidelines: conducting evaluation of dementia and age-related cognitive decline
6. Psychologists must conduct a clinical interview as part of the evaluation
7. Psychologists must be aware that standardized psychological and neuropsychological tests are important tools in the assessment of dementia and age-related cognitive decline
8. When measuring cognitive changes in individuals, psychologists must attempt to estimate premorbid abilities.

9. Psychologists must be sensitive to the limitations and sources of variability and error in psychometric performance
10. Psychologists must recognize that providing constructive feedback, support and education, as well as maintaining a therapeutic alliance, can be important parts of the evaluation process.

Assessment of cognitive functioning among older adults requires specialist training in refined psychometric tools. Psychologists conducting such assessments must learn current diagnostic nomenclature and criteria, gain specialized competence in the selection and use of psychological tests, and understand both the limitations of these tests and the context in which they may be used and interpreted. Assessment of cognitive issues in dementia and age-related cognitive decline is a core focus of the specialty of clinical and neuropsychology. Therefore these guidelines are only intended to suggest the development of an independent proficiency. They are intended to state explicitly some appropriate cautions and concerns for all psychologists who wish to assess cognitive abilities among older adults, particularly when distinguishing between normal and pathological processes.

Address for correspondence

Practice Directorate
American Psychological Association
750 First Street NE
Washington DC 20002-4242
USA

Swedish Consensus on Dementia Diseases

Acta Neurologica Scandinavica (1994) Supplement 157:3

Purpose

This consensus-based document on dementia diseases was developed by dementia researchers in Sweden from 1988 to 1990. It comprises classification and nosology of dementia, the significance of history taking and bedside examination is emphasized and the use of auxiliary diagnostic investigations are discussed (130 references are provided).

Contents

Address for correspondence
Anders Wallin MD PhD
Goteborg University
Department of Clinical Neuroscience
Section of Psychiatry and Neurochemistry
Molndal Hospital
S-43180 Molndal
Sweden

Health Evidence Bulletins

Reference   http://hebw.uwcm.ac.uk/mental/chapter 3.html

Summary

A series of statements concerning dementia with associated evidence.

The statements are:

3.1   Prevention and promotion

a   The *risk factors* for vascular dementia are similar to those for stroke and the scope for prevention is therefore the same. (See Cardiovascular Diseases bulletin in this series.)

b   Some dementing illnesses such as Huntington's disease have specific genetic cause and *genetic counselling* for families at risk should be available.

c   *Public education* is an important area in preparing people to deal with issues associated with dementia.

d   The importance of *aluminium exposure* as a risk factor for Alzheimer's disease is still unknown. While one observational study suggests no significant relationship between aluminium intake (from food, water and medication), an earlier randomized trial of treatment with a metal ion binding compound suggested that there may be a link.

e   Prolonged *postmenopausal hormone replacement therapy (HRT)* delays the onset and reduces the incidence of dementia.

3.2   Diagnosis and assessment

a   *Early identification* and *referral* to specialist services is to be encouraged at the stage when there is a possibility of beneficial intervention, and *multidisciplinary assessment teams* should be utilized.

b   *Simple mental state tests* are adequate to provide diagnosis in primary care and routine investigation before referral is unwarranted. The probability of dementia was greatly reduced with normal serial 7s, seven-digit span, recall of three items or clock drawing (likelihood ratio, LR, 0.06–0.2). Abnormal clock drawing increased the likelihood of Alzheimer's disease as distinguished from other dementias (LR 3.7; 95% CI 2.4–5.9) and normal drawing decreased the likelihood (LR 0.03; CI 0.01–0.07).

c   Ready access to *appropriate investigations* should be available to patients.

d   *Reversible dementia* is now very rare (<1%) and mostly metabolic, toxic, neurosurgical or psychiatric (depressive) in origin.

e   Appropriate *training and education* should be provided to professionals who care for patients with dementia as this is likely to be beneficial.

3.3   Treatment and care

a   The following strategies are recommended for the care of patients with dementia:
- *Early treatment* of reversible dementia
- Maintaining the *physical health and fitness* of patients
- *Appropriate drug* treatment of associated psychosis
- *Active management* of acute illness
- *Local day and sitter support*
- *Reminiscence techniques*
- Highly flexible *respite care*
- *Training* in the management of wandering and unsafe behaviour.

b   *Behavioural management* is likely to be beneficial. One small study suggested that occupational therapy was of value for long-term geriatric patients with slight to moderate dementia.

c   Planning and design of patients' *living environment* is likely to be helpful.

d   In a trial of dementia care in nursing homes, the *AGE dementia care programme* (Activities, Guidelines for psychotropic medications and Educational rounds) reduced the prevalence of behaviour disorders and the use of antipsychotic drugs and restraints.

e   Formal *reality orientation sessions* and *validation therapy* are of uncertain value.

f   *Physical restraints* should not be used.

3.4   Specific drug therapies

a   *Neuroleptics* have a consistent modest effect in agitated patients. No drug takes precedence.

b   Long-term treatment with *acetyl.l.carnitine* may produce a deceleration in decline of patients with dementia.

c   The use of *hydergine* has not yet proven to be of benefit in the treatment of Alzheimer's dementia, but might be of some limited use in vascular dementia. A systematic review is in preparation.

d   There is no convincing evidence at present that *nimodipine* is a useful treatment for dementia, but review is not yet complete.

e   At this stage, the evidence does not support the use of *piracetam* in the treatment of people with dementia or cognitive impairment.

f   Although the evidence for a beneficial effect of *selegiline* on patients with Alzheimer's disease is promising, there is not yet enough evidence to recommend its use routinely in practice.

g   A review provides no convincing evidence that high-dose *tacrine* is a useful treatment for the symptoms of Alzheimer's disease.

h   *Glycosaminoglycan* was found to be superior to placebo in a multicentre double-blind trial in the treatment of the earliest manifestations of a dementing process.

i   *Nicergoline* is superior to placebo in treating multi-infarct dementia.

j   Further *Cochrane reviews* of drug therapies are in progress.

k   An initial randomized controlled trial suggested that *donepezil* probably produces an improvement corresponding to 'turning the clock back' by 3–6 months (equivalent to a gain of about 0.05 to 0.08 QALYs), but that the benefits were small and the weight of evidence unconvincing. The results of further ongoing studies are awaited.

l   Psychotherapeutic interventions are of little help to patients, but may be of help to carers.

3.5   Rehabilitation and continuing care

a   *24-hour support services* should be available.

b   Efforts to reduce *carers' stress* are beneficial. A programme of patient and caregiver training, with long-term follow-up, suggested statistically significant (but not huge) increases in survival and time spent at home. A review is due soon.

c   The following strategies are likely to be beneficial in the care of patients with dementia:
   - *Formal care planning* with identified key workers
   - Maximizing the use of *remaining abilities*
   - *Regular reviews* and continuing *backup*
   - Maintaining sufferer in the *most appropriate place*
   - *Timely referral* to new services to match changing services
   - *Joint planning of care* between health and social services and voluntary agencies
   - *Advice to carers* on financial and other services
   - *Support to carers* through pre- and post-death grief
   - Provision of specialist services for *younger sufferers*.

3.6   Prognosis – length of survival

a   There is a clear relationship between severity of dementia and survival time. The combination of wandering, falling and behavioural problems is associated with shorter survival.

Address for correspondence

Dr Alison Weightman
Protocol Enhancement Project
Duthie Library
UWCM
Cardiff CF4 4XN
Wales

weightmanal@cardiff.ac.uk

Epidemiologically Based Needs Assessment: Alzheimer's Disease and Other Dementias

Reference   Melzer D, Pearce K, Cooper B, Brayne C In Stevens A, Raftery J, Mant J, eds *Health Care Needs Assessment: The Epidemiologically Based Needs Assessment Reviews – 1st Series Update.* Abingdon: Radcliffe Medical Press (in press)

Purpose

A revised edition of a systematic literature review examining the effectiveness of treatments, models of care and services available for people with dementia. One of a series of evidence based reviews commissioned by the UK NHS Executive. The current version of this text may be further revised and updated before eventual publication.

Summary

The bulk of the review consists of three chapters to discuss services and resources currently available; effectiveness of treatments and interventions; and models of care – towards rationally based services for dementia. There are brief chapters on health information systems; research and development (especially outcome measures); and future directions for research, service provision and policy in the area of dementia.

Services currently available

These are outlined according to the main providers, namely primary care, local authority social services departments, old age psychiatry services, geriatric medicine and other hospital specialties. Requirements for good services are listed and many of the problems of existing provision are discussed.

Effectiveness of treatments and services

These are discussed under three headings according to the stage of dementia.

1. Before clinical onset of dementia:

- No measures are proven to be effective for primary prevention of dementia, though steps to reduce cerebrovascular disease and trauma may be important.
- General population screening for dementia is not indicated.
- Clinical recognition of established dementia should be improved.
- Genetic testing is currently only indicated in families with several members affected by early onset dementia.

2. In mild to moderate dementia:

- The diagnosis is essentially a clinical one, augmented where appropriate with investigations; much of the diagnosis and management can be conducted in primary care.
- Anticholinesterase drugs offer 2 to 4 point improvement on the ADAS-COG scale over 6 months in trials.
- Neuroleptic drugs show small but significant effects in controlling behaviour and psychological symptoms, but side effects and overprescribing are common.
- Psychological and behavioural therapies are promising but good evidence from trials is in short supply.
- Organizational approaches to improving care co-ordination can be effective.
- Respite care services are popular with carers, but there is little evidence from trials that respite reduces carer stress or time to institutionalization.
- Support groups can delay institutionalization.

3. In moderate to severe dementia:

- Supportive and practical care needs predominate.
- Social care 'case management' can be effective in supporting older people, including those with dementia.
- Quality of care in institutional settings needs improvement.
- Standards of care for people with cognitive impairment admitted to acute hospitals are in great need of improvement.

Models of care

There is insufficient evidence on which to base a quantified model of resources and care for dementia. Key elements would include:

- Central role of primary care for most diagnosis, information, management of medication and co-existing illness, referral and monitoring.
- Meeting informal caregiver needs for information and practical support.
- Integrated secondary health and social care provision, preferably in multidisciplinary teams.
- Important role of specialist old age psychiatry services, particularly for those with complex problems, including challenging behaviour.
- Improving care for people with dementia in acute hospital settings.
- Active programmes to improve care in institutional

settings, including managing medication and physical illness, and active measures to improve quality of life.

- Adequate continuing care provision within the NHS for dementia associated with severe behaviour disorder and/or physical illness, combined with an equitable system of cost coverage for community support services and long-term residential care.

Future directions

These will be governed by three main requirements:

- Careful testing and appraisal of new research findings and emerging technologies.
- Improvement in the quality and provision of existing services for those with a clinical degree of dementia.
- Methods for earlier detection, diagnosis and treatment to combat the disease process at an earlier stage and prevent or delay its progression.

Further references

The review contains 212 references up to 1998.

Address for correspondence

D Melzer
Department of Public Health & Primary Care
Institute of Public Health,
Forvie Site,
Robinson Way,
Cambridge CB2 2SR
UK

dm214@medschl.cam.ac.uk

Differential Diagnosis of Dementing Diseases: National Institutes of Health Consensus Development Program 63

References   NIH (1987) *Differential Diagnosis of Dementing Diseases.* NIH Consensus Statement Online 6: 1–27

NIH (1988) *Alzheimer's Disease and Associated Disorders* 2: 4–15

Purpose

To assess the current state of knowledge about the differential diagnosis of the dementias. The result is a summary following $1\frac{1}{2}$ days of presentations by experts from relevant fields and by public organizations involved with dementias. A consensus panel consisted of representatives from neurology, psychiatry, geriatric medicine, epidemiology, psychology, family practice, neuropathology, nursing and the public.

Summary

Five questions were considered:

1. What is dementia?
2. What are the dementing diseases and which of them can readily be arrested or reversed?
3. What should be included in the initial evaluation of dementia?
4. What diagnostic tests should be performed, and when are these tests indicated?
5. What are the priorities for future research on diagnosing the dementias?

What diagnostic tests should be performed, and when are these tests indicated?

The best diagnostic test is a careful history and physical and mental status examination by a physician with a knowledge of and interest in dementia and the dementing diseases. Such an evaluation is time consuming, but nothing else can replace it. Sub-specialty consultation proves helpful in selected cases.

The laboratory tests that are used should be individualized based on the history and physical and mental status examination. Over-testing may expose the patient to discomfort, inconvenience, excess costs, and the likelihood of false positive tests that may lead to additional unnecessary testing. Under-testing also has hazards, for example in elderly persons, where medical diseases may have non-specific presentations such as dementia.

All patients with new onset of dementia should have several basic and standard diagnostic studies, with modifications to be made according to individual circumstances:

- complete blood count
- electrolyte panel
- screening metabolic panel
- thyroid function tests
- Vitamin B_{12} and folate levels
- tests for syphilis and, depending on history, for human immunodeficiency antibodies
- urinalysis
- electrocardiogram
- chest X-ray

Most of the readily reversible metabolic, endocrine, deficiency and infectious states, whether causative or complicating, will be revealed by these simple investigations when combined with history and physical examination.

Other ancillary studies are appropriate in certain common situations:

1. Computed tomography of the brain (without contrast) is appropriate in the presence of history suggestive of a mass, or focal neurologic signs, or in dementia of brief duration. Unless such diagnosis is obvious on first contact, computed tomography should be done.
2. All medications that are not absolutely necessary should be discontinued.
3. Electroencephalograms are appropriate for patients with altered consciousness or suspected seizures, depending on the clinical circumstances.
4. Formal psychiatric assessment is desirable when depression is suspected.
5. Inpatient hospitalization should be considered when the history is unclear, if the patient is suicidal, when an acute deterioration has occurred without apparent cause, or if the social situation precludes adequate observation.
6. Neuropsychological evaluation is appropriate (a) to obtain baseline information against which to measure change in cases in which diagnosis is in doubt; (b) before and following treatment; (c) in cases of exceptionally bright individuals suspected of early dementia; (d) in cases of ambiguous imaging findings that require elucidation; (e) to help distinguish dementia from depression and delirium; and (f) to provide additional information about the extent and nature of impairment following focal or multifocal brain injury.

7. Speech and language analysis can be very helpful. In some patients, complex language disorders can simulate dementia; in others, the skilful speech pathologist can help the patient and family to communicate better.

The role of other studies is controversial, and firm rules for their routine use are not appropriate. Undue weight should not be placed on isolated laboratory findings unless they are consistent with previous clinical information. Examples of these other studies include the following:

1. Magnetic resonance imaging. This is more sensitive than computed tomography for detection of small infarcts, mass lesions, atrophy of the brainstem and other subcortical structures; it also may clarify ambiguous computed tomography findings. Inexperienced interpreters may make too much of ambiguous or non-specific findings on magnetic resonance imaging.
2. Regional cerebral blood flow and metabolism measurements (positron emission tomography and single photon emission computed tomography). These are research techniques that have no proven *routine* clinical value at the present time. Their value in predicting Huntington's and Alzheimer's disease in individuals at risk is under investigation.
3. Lumbar puncture. This is not routinely required in the initial evaluation of dementia. It should be performed when other clinical findings suggest an active infection or vasculitis. At present, cerebrospinal fluid markers for Alzheimer's disease are not sufficiently well developed to justify routine lumbar puncture.
4. Electrophysiological techniques such as event-related potentials that are recorded using special electro-encephalographic techniques. These are not recommended for routine use.
5. Brain biopsy for non-tumorous and non-infectious diseases. This is rarely justified except in a small number of unusual clinical situations.
6. Biological markers for progressive degenerative dementing diseases. These are still in the investigative stage. Although some give promise, they are not ready for widespread or routine use.
7. Significant major findings have been made on the molecular genetics of conditions like Huntington's and Alzheimer's diseases, but these findings have restricted usefulness at present.
8. Carotid ultrasound. This is of no value except sometimes in the search for the cause of infarcts.

What are the priorities for future research on diagnosing the dementias?

Diagnosis of the dementing diseases has improved over the past 10 years. Nevertheless, there is room for improvement in accuracy of diagnosis. Advances in genetics and molecular biology have opened the door to new areas of research, but are not immediately applicable to clinical diagnosis. While awaiting the development of definitive *in vivo* diagnostic tests, it is necessary to rely on autopsy correlation and validation. These remain essential for studies concerned with the search for diagnostic markers, neuropsychological findings, neuroimaging results, outcome of clinical therapeutic trials, and delineation of clinical–pathologic syndromes. Although it is impossible to list all the approaches to future research that may prove fruitful, the panel recommends that highest priority should go to research on the following:

1. Exploration of potential biological diagnostic markers, innovative as well as logical extensions of ongoing research, with special emphasis on families with autopsy-diagnosed dementias.
2. Evaluation of neuroimaging by long-term follow-up of patients, correlation with clinical and neuropsychologic findings, and tissue histopathology. Families with autopsy-diagnosed dementias should be given special attention.
3. Evaluation of results obtained with current neuropsychologic instruments in populations that differ in age, education, ethnic composition and social or cultural background, using long-term follow-up and correlation with clinical, neuroimaging and neuropathologic findings.
4. Assessment of the role of vascular disease in dementia by combining clinical, neuropsychologic, neuroimaging and neuropathologic findings as well as by examining vascular risk factors.
5. Investigation of neuropsychologic test profiles characteristic of specific dementias and validation by means of clinical, neuroimaging and neuropathologic findings.
6. Design of multivariate studies to determine the optimal combination of diagnostic strategies, including elements of the history and physical examination, mental status and specialized tests needed to differentiate the dementias common in each age group.
7. Investigation of the mechanisms by which various drugs, non-psychoactive as well as psychoactive, induce or precipitate a dementia syndrome.
8. Exploration of the mechanisms by which depression induces or precipitates a dementia syndrome.
9. Investigation of the less common degenerative diseases, such as Pick's disease, progressive supranuclear palsy, olivopontocerebellar degeneration and progressive subcortical gliosis.

Conclusion

Dementia is a clinical state, diagnosable only by clinical methods. Every patient with dementia deserves precise assessment, not only of the fact of dementia, but of the manifestations and the manner in which the disability is produced. Dementia can be caused by a multitude of different dementing diseases, some of which are arrestable or reversible, and many of which are preventable.

The first approach to a patient with suspected dementia is a careful clinical evaluation. A laboratory test, whether chemical, biological, imaging or psychological, should never be used as a substitute for the physician's time, expertise and clinical judgment. Because dementia is primarily a behavioral diagnosis, the initial medical evaluation should include an assessment of how well the patient functions in his or her daily life as well as a family history and neurological and standardized mental status examinations. Relatives, friends and neighbours often can provide information especially valuable in assessing a patient suspected of having dementia.

The diagnosis of dementia has become more accurate over the past 10 years, but thorough assessment still cannot be done rapidly. Because serious implications are inherent in making a diagnosis of irreversible dementia and in missing any conditions that may be arrested or reversed, physicians are used to take the time necessary to make this thorough evaluation and to refer patients to specialists when they want further confirmation of clinical findings.

Because large gaps still exist in current knowledge on the diagnosis of dementia, the panel has made specific recommendations for further research that will result in improving the differential diagnosis of dementing diseases.

Screening for Cognitive Impairment in the Elderly

References Patterson C (1994) Screening for cognitive impairment in the elderly. In: *Canadian Task Force on the Periodic Health Examination. Canadian Guide to Clinical Preventive Health Care*, pp. 902–9. (Updated version in the *Canadian Medical Association Journal* (1991) 144: 425–31)

www.ctfphc.org/Abstracts_printable/Ch75abs.htm

Purpose

To make recommendations about screening for cognitive impairment among asymptomatic elderly persons in Canada, updating a 1991 report.

Summary

Despite the theoretical advantages of identifying individuals with cognitive impairment, there is no evidence to indicate whether this leads to a net benefit or risk to the individual. Although pharmaceutical agents are able to produce measurable changes in cognitive performance in people with Alzheimer's disease, none has been shown to result consistently in clinically significant improvement. The high cost of investigation to exclude reversible causes of dementia and the negative effects of labeling are examples of potential harm.

Identification of asymptomatic cognitively impaired individuals by the use of short mental status tests or by any other means has not been demonstrated to produce benefit. Thus there is insufficient evidence to recommend for or against screening. The prudent physician should be alert for any reports or behavior which may indicate cognitive impairment (e.g. forgetting appointments, poor medication compliance), and then pursue appropriate strategies for further investigation and treatment.

Unanswered questions (research agenda)

1. Although two of the brief mental status instruments reviewed appear satisfactory for case finding in primary care, they are not ideal, and more sensitive specific instruments are desirable.
2. The search for effective treatments for Alzheimer's disease should incorporate outcome measures including physical functioning, behavior measures of caregiver burden and ability to delay or prevent institutional care.
3. Trials of screening are necessary to examine the impact of detecting cognitive impairment, its subsequent investigation and treatment.
4. Studies should be directed towards discovering any negative effects from attaching the label of Alzheimer's disease or cognitive impairment to a person.

Address for correspondence

Christopher Patterson
Professor and Head
Division of Geriatric Medicine
McMaster University
Hamilton
Ontario
Canada

Practice Parameter for Diagnosis and Evaluation of Dementia

Reference   Quality Standards Subcommittee of the American Academy of Neurology (1994) Report. *Neurology* 44: 2203–6

Purpose

The Quality Standards Subcommittee of the American Academy of Neurology is charged with development and practice parameters and the document outlines what the subcommittee believe to be the most useful components of the diagnostic evaluation of elderly patients with cognitive complaints suggesting dementia.

Summary

The recommendations have been designated standards, guidelines and options according to the following criteria.

Definitions. Classification of evidence

Class I. Evidence provided by one or more well-designed randomized controlled clinical trials.

Class II. Evidence provided by one or more well-designed clinical studies such as case–control studies, cohort studies and so forth.

Class III. Evidence provided by expert opinion, non-randomized historical controls, or one or more case reports.

Strength of recommendations

Standards. Generally accepted principles for patient management that reflect a high degree of clinical certainty (i.e. based on Class I evidence or, when circumstances preclude randomized clinical trials, overwhelming evidence from Class II studies that directly addresses the question at hand, or from decision analysis that directly addresses all the issues.

Guidelines. Recommendations for patient management that may identify a particular strategy or range of management strategies and that reflect moderate clinical certainty (i.e. based on Class II evidence that directly addresses the issue, or strong consensus of Class III evidence.

Practice options or advisories. Other strategies for patient management for which there is unclear clinical certainty (i.e. based on inconclusive or conflicting evidence or opinion). Practice options in certain clinical situations may be considered medically indicated.

Practice parameters. Results in the form of one or more specific recommendations, from a scientifically-based analysis of a specific clinical problem.

Recommendations

The parameters are based on an extensive search of the literature culminating in 110 articles used to prepare the document. The main headings for the paper are Identification of Dementia, Diagnostic Workup, Differential Diagnosis, Identification of Dementia.

Guidelines

Individuals who should be evaluated for evidence of dementia should include those with memory or other cognitive complaints, with or without functional impairment, elderly patients in whom there is a question of incompetency, depressed or anxious patients with cognitive complaints, and patients who arouse suspicion of cognitive impairment during their interview despite the absence of complaints.

Cognitive or mental status testing should include assessment of level of arousal, attention, orientation, recent remote memory, language, praxis, visuospatial function, calculations and judgement.

Options

If there are changes in intellectual function, the patients do not meet the criteria for dementia. Re-evaluation after 6–12 months may help document cognitive decline.

Detailed neuropsychological testing is often valuable to detect subtle cognitive difficulties. Standardized instruments may assess the clinician in diagnosis, particularly tests of cognitive function.

Diagnostic workup

The neurological history and examination, including mental state examination, are essential components of the standard diagnostic workup with dementia. Diagnostic tests are also necessary in the differential diagnosis of dementia to rule out metabolic and structural causes. A lumbar puncture should be performed when any of the following are present – metastatic cancer, suspicion of CNS infection, reactive serum syphilis urology, hydrocephalus, dementia in a person under the age of 55, a rapidly progressing or unusual dementia, immunosuppression, or suspicion of CNS vasculitis.

Detailed workup should include full blood count, electrolytes including calcium, glucose, renal function tests, liver function tests, thyroid function tests, vitamin B_{12}, syphilis serology; not recommended routinely are sedimentation rate, folate level, HIV testing, chest X-ray, urine analysis, 24-hour urine collection for heavy metals, toxicology screen, neuroimaging study (CT or MRI), neuropsychological testing, lumbar puncture, EEG, PET scan and SPET scan.

Detailed neuropsychological testing may be performed; EEG may be of assistance in distinguishing depression or delirium from dementia and in suspected encephalitis seizures, metabolic encephalopathy, or Creutzfeldt-Jakob disease.

Differential diagnosis

Use of clinical criteria with a diagnosis of Alzheimer's disease. The ischaemic score may be used to diagnose vascular dementia.

Address for correspondence

Joanne F Okagaki
American Academy of Neurology
Suite 335
2221 University Avenue SE
Minneapolis, MN 55414
USA

Consensus Statement on the Assessment and Investigation of an Elderly Person with Suspected Cognitive Impairment by a Specialist Old Age Psychiatry Service

Reference   The Royal College of Psychiatrists (1995) *Council Report CR49* (currently being updated)

Purpose

The document is a statement from the specialist Section of Old Age Psychiatry from the UK Royal College of Psychiatrists concerning acceptable service practice. It was developed following extensive and lengthy discussion and a nationwide exercise involving feedback, locally led discussions, pilot project and audits. It is accepted that the minimum standard should only be accepted when a service is resourced to Royal College recommended levels of staffing. The document is primarily intended to provide guidance and advice to purchasers of services, but also to assist service providers with consideration of their own practice, with particular reference to training.

Summary

There should be easier referral access and responsiveness.
    Practice is described under a number of headings:

1. *The assessment process.* Home assessment; medical assessment; collateral history; mental state assessment; physical examination; aggravating factors; diagnosis
2. *Service characteristics.* Comprehensiveness; communication; geriatric liaison; further assessment
3. *Clinical investigation.* Practicalities; appropriate investigation. This section, unlike the others, has definite recommendations.

There is insufficient firm evidence to allow authoritative recommendations in the definitive list of investigations. The Consensus includes the following: *blood tests*: full blood count; ESR; B_{12} and folate; thyroid function tests; Urea and electrolytes; calcium liver function test and glucose. Tests for *syphilis* are recommended to be carried out unless the clinical picture is 'typical' (not further defined). *Urine analysis, electrocardiogram, chest X-ray* should be carried out unless the clinical picture is typical and there are no significant cardiovascular or respiratory signs. *Computed tomography* scan should be performed if practical unless the history goes back for longer than a year and there is a typical clinical picture. Consideration of age should not influence the decision. *Immunology* should be carried out if the possibility of a cerebral autoimmune disease is present. *Normal pressure hydrocephalus* assessment should be pursued unless the triad of features are not present. *Neuropsychology* should be carried out; it may be helpful, particularly with early cases.

Address for correspondence

Royal College of Psychiatrists
17 Belgrave Square
London SW1X 9PG
UK

Diagnosis and Treatment of Alzheimer's Disease and Related Disorders

References   Small GW, Rabins PV, Barry PP *et al* (1997) Consensus Statement of the American Association for Geriatric Psychiatry, the Alzheimer's Association and the American Geriatrics Society. *Journal of the American Medical Association* 278: 1363–71

Purpose

This followed a consensus conference held in January 1997. The target audience was primary care physicians, and seven questions were addressed:

1. How prevalent is Alzheimer's disease (AD), and what are its risk factors and its impact on society?
2. What are the different forms of dementia and how can they be recognized?
3. What constitutes safe and effective treatment for AD? What are the indications and contraindications of specific treatments?
4. What management strategies are available to the primary care practitioner?
5. What are the available medical specialty and community resources?
6. What are the important policy issues, and how can policy makers improve access to care for dementia patients?
7. What are the most promising questions for future research?

Summary

1. Dementia and AD, its most common form, incur substantial costs to society. The diagnosis of AD, moreover, continues to be missed in clinical practice. Alzheimer's disease is under-reported and unrecognized because many patients do not seek evaluation and family members tend to compensate for deficits. In addition, physicians may fail to recognize the early signs of disease or to diagnose the disorder correctly, even though effective treatment and management techniques are available to enhance quality of life. The lack of a specific diagnostic test for AD means that physicians must conduct a focused clinical assessment and informant interview on patients with suspected AD.

2. The diagnosis of AD is primarily one of inclusion, and the diagnosis can usually be made using standardized clinical criteria. As many patients do not visit a physician for the treatment of suspected dementia at the time of diagnosis, but rather for another medical problem, physicians should be alert to concerns about cognitive decline and evaluate promptly. Progressive memory and other cognitive impairment in a clear state of consciousness is most commonly indicative of AD. Vascular dementia may be overdiagnosed, but its progression is potentially preventable if risk factors for stroke are recognized and treatment is initiated.

3. While AD is a complex disorder that ultimately may require treatment by a neurologist, geriatrician or geriatric psychiatrist, much of its treatment can be managed successfully in the primary care setting. Longitudinal monitoring of therapies and regular health maintenance checkups are essential. New cognitive and functional enhancers may improve memory and other aspects of cognition and function. Emotional and behavior disturbances can be treated and their resolution can provide significant improvement in quality of life. All psychopharmacologic therapies should be used judiciously in the elderly.

4. Family intervention is critical. Education, counseling and support can help caregivers cope with feelings of anger, frustration and guilt in response to a patient's sometimes provocative behavior. Family members benefit from reassurance that their responses are common. Relatives' anxiety about their own memory lapses may respond to counseling, coupled with a neuropsychological evaluation. In some cases, such assessments uncover early symptoms of disease, allowing for prompt treatment and management.

5. Newly evolving delivery systems and reimbursement practices are exacerbating the nation's inadequate and fragmented system of care. Better definition of quality care, based on rigorous quantitative data, will enable policymakers and delivery systems to create new approaches to ensure access to essential medical, psychosocial and community resources. Given the morbidity and mortality associated with AD, increasing expenditures are essential to fill an already critical medical and social need.

6. Answers to a variety of research questions will help resolve these issues. Investigators need to focus on barriers to care and conduct longitudinal studies, using both naturalistic and treatment-based designs. Cost-effectiveness needs to be assessed for both diagnostic and treatment approaches.

Address for correspondence

Gary Small
University of California at Los Angeles
Neuropsychiatric Institute and Hospital
760 Westwood Plaza, Room 37–432
Los Angeles, CA 90241759, USA

Screening for Dementia

References Atkins D for the US Preventive Services Task Force (1996) *Guide to Clinical Preventive Services*, 2nd edn. Williams and Wilkins 531–40

Summary

There is insufficient evidence to recommend for or against routine screening for dementia in asymptomatic elderly persons. Clinicians should periodically ask patients about their functional status at home and at work, and they should remain alert to changes in performance with age. When possible, information about daily activities should be solicited from family members or other persons. Brief tests such as the MMSE should be used to assess cognitive function in patients in whom the suspicion of dementia is raised by restrictions in daily activities, concerns of family members, or other evidence of worsening function (e.g. trouble with finances, medications, transportation). Possible effects of education and cultural differences should be considered when interpreting results of cognitive tests. The diagnosis of dementia should not be based on results of screening tests alone. Patients suspected of having dementia should be examined for other causes of changing mental status, including depression, delirium, medication effects and coexisting medical illnesses.

Dementia Identification and Assessment: Guidelines for Primary Care Practitioners

Reference   US Dept of Veterans Affairs & University Health System Consortium. March 1997

Purpose
To provide guidelines for the identification and assessment of dementia in primary care

Summary
This guideline provides an algorithm for the differential diagnosis of dementia. By following this algorithm the specific sub type of dementia can be identified. The treatment of dementia from both a non-pharmacological and pharmacological point of view is outlined in the guideline and a section on the caregiver is also included. The non-pharmacological interventions that are included relate to change in home environment, training for caregivers, advice for caregivers regarding diet and hydration and how to prevent skin breakdown, and directions on bladder and bowel routines. The guideline also deals with the treatment of underlying diseases such as cerebrovascular disease, Parkinson's disease and normal pressure hydrocephalus together with the treatment of toxic and metabolic causes of dementia.

A summary of the pharmacological treatments of behavioural and psychological symptoms in dementia is also included, as is a discussion on the use of cholinesterase inhibitors for cognitive symptoms.

Address for correspondence
University Health System Consortium (UHC) 2001, Spring Road, Suite 700, Oak Brook, IL 60523 USA

Early identification of Alzheimer's disease and related dementias

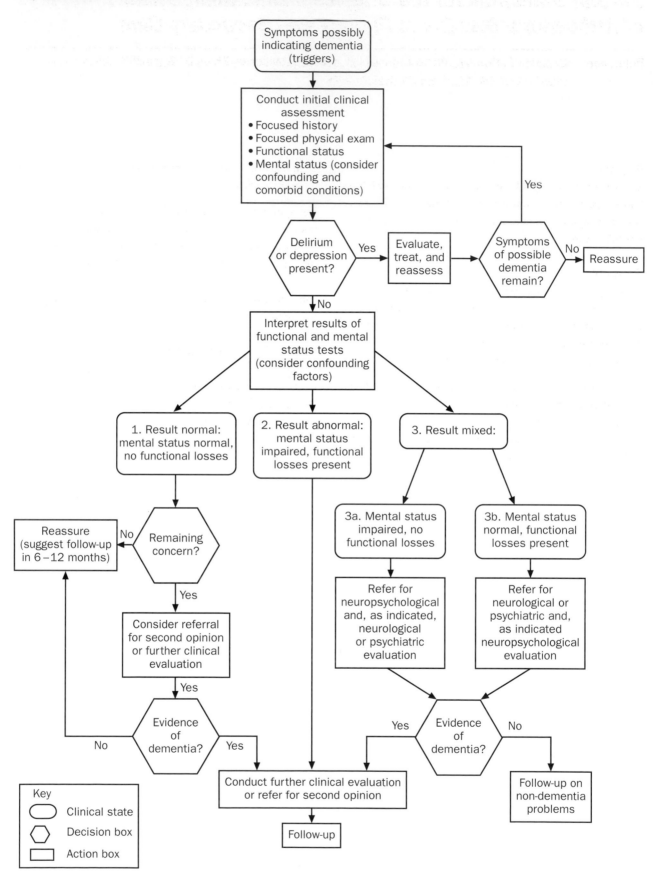

Setting Standards for the Diagnosis and Management of Alzheimer's Disease in Primary and Secondary Care

Reference   Banerjee S, Burns A, Clubb A, Jones R, Lawlor B, Rossor M, Sharp D, Wilcock G, Wilkinson D (1997) *Geriatric Medicine Clinical Bulletin*

Purpose

To overcome the difficulty in diagnosis and general lack of knowledge and treatment which are obstacles to effective Alzheimer's disease management in both primary and secondary care.

Summary

Areas highlighted included summary boxes for key symptoms, the exclusion of reversible causes with suggested tests and the role of neuroimaging, and exclusion of non-dementia causes – delirium and depression.

Key symptoms of Alzheimer's disease include:

- an insidious onset of symptoms, initially memory loss in most cases which progresses over time
- emergence of aphasia
- agnosia (failure of recognition, particularly obvious with failure to recognize carers and relations)
- apraxia (inability to carry out motor tasks despite intact motor and sensory function).

Key symptoms of vascular dementia, dementia with Lewy bodies, and a note of other dementias are also given.

Alzheimer's disease management includes a note of treatment recommendations, the use of support services and the importance of follow-up, both in terms of continuity of care and assessment of the effect of drug treatments.

Address for correspondence

Professor Alistair Burns
Academic Department of Old Age Psychiatry
Withington Hospital
Manchester M20 8LR
UK

Assessing Older People with Dementia Living in the Community

Reference Social Services Inspectorate Report of the SSI workshop and visits (1995) *Practical Issues for Social and Health Services.* UK Department of Health

Purpose

To improve the knowledge base and inform the day-to-day practice of operational staff and their managers, helping them to develop a multidisciplinary approach to the assessment and care management of older people with dementia living in the community. It comes from a survey which took place in five local authorities in 1995, and is based on semi-structured interviews with operational social services and health staff, both purchasers and providers, who are developing joint working services for older people with dementia. The information is based on professional practice, not scientific research. Four action checklists are provided, which address the key issues highlighted by the project report and are intended for use by all those who may be in contact with or responsible for assessing older people with dementia.

Summary

See checklists.

Address for correspondence

Department of Health
PO Box 410
Wetherby LS23 7LN
UK

Action checklist 1: Taking responsibility for older people with dementia

With early, informed social and health care assessment and appropriate support, older people with dementia can maintain their independence and quality of life in the community. Checklist 1 will help all those with a responsibility for meeting care management objectives for older people with dementia – including SSD older persons and mental health services, and primary and community health services – to understand the local context and to ensure co-ordinated policies and responses.

✓ Are the likely numbers known of older people with dementia in the locality, both living alone and with family carers?
✓ Do assessors understand how dementia affects older people and their ability to communicate and make judgments?
✓ Are the numbers and needs of older people from minority ethnic communities known?
✓ Are older people with dementia offered the same opportunities to make choices and decisions about their lives as other community care users?

✓ Do social and health services agencies share aims, standards and priorities for services for older people with dementia?
✓ Are joint aspirations for older people with dementia enshrined in the community care plan and in joint policy statements/commissioning strategies?
✓ Are elected members aware of and committed to meeting the needs of older people with dementia?
✓ Are housing agencies and independent sector organizations involved in planning strategies for older people with dementia?
✓ Have authorities considered how to involve users as well as carers in planning service strategies for older people with dementia?
✓ Is joint training available to develop a common understanding of dementia and shared standards and aims for providing community care for this group of older people?

Action checklist 2: Developing multi-agency working for older people with dementia

A co-ordinated approach to identifying and assessing the needs of older people who may have dementia is essential. Checklist 2 will help practitioners and their managers to build links and work effectively across professional and organizational boundaries.

✓ Have different models/structures (multi-agency teams, resource centres) for joint working been explored in the context of local circumstances/organizational systems?

✓ Are voluntary/independent sector organization staff and volunteers involved in assessment and care planning for older people with dementia?

✓ Are housing agencies involved in assessment and care planning for older people with dementia?

✓ Are the respective roles in the assessment and care planning process of health and social services staff clearly set out and understood?

✓ Are GP practices/primary health care teams provided with information about community care assessment procedures and services?

✓ Do social services and health services staff have informal, routine communication about assessment/intervention?

✓ Are information systems/records easily accessed between GP practices and SSDs?

✓ Is joint training available for social and health care staff?

✓ Have linkworker or attached social worker schemes been considered?

✓ Are referral systems co-ordinated between social work staff and the GP, community psychiatric nurse and psychogeriatrician?

✓ Are community care and care programme approach systems integrated as far as possible?

Action checklist 3: Assessing older people with dementia

The nature of dementia requires particular skills and knowledge in order to ensure that quality assessment is achieved. Checklist 3 will help front-line staff ensure that dementia is identified at an early stage, that presenting problems are handled appropriately, and that referrals are made to relevant specialist services where necessary.

Information and identification

✓ Is information available in appropriate places/formats so that users and their family/friends (including black and minority ethnic people) can access assessment and services?

✓ Do procedures exist to ensure early identification of older people with dementia?

✓ Do community care assessment forms include trigger questions to help assessors recognize dementia?

✓ Have health and social services agreed who (e.g. social worker, community psychiatric nurse) can carry out an assessment?

✓ Can assessors recognize signs of mild to severe dementia in older people?

✓ Do assessors seek advice/refer appropriately in order to distinguish between dementia and other conditions (e.g. depression) producing similar behaviour?

✓ Do social workers recognize the health needs of older people with dementia?

✓ Are 75+ health checks routinely offered to screen for dementia?

✓ Are older people with suspected dementia referred for specialist diagnosis and medical check?

Communication and risk assessment

✓ Do social workers and other assessors have the necessary communication skills to work with older people with dementia?

✓ Do social workers and other assessors have sufficient time to work with an older person to develop understanding and trust, and to ensure thorough, responsive assessment?

✓ Is a diagnosis of dementia explained to users as well as to carers?

✓ Are independent advocates (including minority ethnic advocates) available to help older people with dementia put forward their views?

✓ Are the needs of older people with dementia who have other disabilities/sensory loss taken into account?

✓ Are the needs of the carer identified and taken account of in the assessment and care plan?

✓ Is information sought as appropriate from "indirect" carers, friends and neighbours to help build up a picture of the individual?

✓ Do authorities have policies and procedures to support older people with dementia to accept reasonable risks?

✓ Do practitioners understand the use of guardianship under the Mental Health Act?

✓ Do policies and procedures on abuse of adults/older people encompass the needs of older people with dementia?

Action checklist 4: Care planning and review

Although this project focused primarily on assessment, the boundaries between assessment, care planning, service provision and review are not clear-cut. Checklist 4 will help practitioners to consider appropriate care planning and service provision and review for older people with dementia.

✓ Are appropriate arrangements in place for continuous assessment, monitoring and review of older people with dementia?

✓ Are the needs of the older person and carer separately acknowledged?

✓ Do assessment/review techniques focus on positive/possible achievements of older people with dementia?

✓ Does each older person with dementia have a key worker?

✓ Are there local community specialist (resource/day centres) services for older people with dementia?

✓ Do specialist services for older people with dementia meet the cultural needs of minority ethnic older people?

✓ Do specialist services for older people with dementia meet the specific needs of those with sensory impairment, multiple disability and/or multiple health problems?

Diagnosis and Management of Alzheimer's Disease and Other Disorders Associated with Dementia: The Role of Neurologists in Europe

Reference   Waldemar G, Dubois B, Emre M, Scheltens P, Tariska P, Rossor M (2000) Diagnosis and management of Alzheimer's disease and other disorders associated with dementia. The role of neurologists in Europe. European Federation of Neurological Societies. *European Journal of Neurology* 7: 133–44.

Purpose

A task force was set up in 1988 to develop guidelines for diagnostic evaluation and treatment of dementia by the European Federation of Neurological Societies (EFNS) scientific panel on dementia. The aim of the task force was to provide evidence-based recommendations and to highlight the role of neurologists in the management of patients with Alzheimer's disease and other disorders associated with dementia.

Summary

The recommendations were based on a review of available evidence-based guidelines supplemented with further literature reviews. They were derived from consensus meetings and relate to individual patient management.

The particular contributions of neurologists include: early identification and differential diagnosis of rare and uncommon brain disorders causing cognitive and behavioural symptoms; referral for interpretation of ancillary investigations; and identification and treatment of vascular and other concurrent factors in dementia. It is recommended that neurologists should have a clear role in the management of dementia in Europe. They should be involved in diagnostic evaluation of dementia and facilitate the development of multidisciplinary teams for evaluation and management of patients with cognitive disturbances. The increasing role of neurology in the management of patients with dementia has important implications for training and education.

Recommendations

The neurologist should be involved in the diagnostic evaluation of patients with dementia.

Cognitive assessment is central to diagnosis and management of dementias.

Quantitative neuropsychology exploring individual cognitive domains with validated tests of graded difficulty is very powerful. However, it is not routinely available throughout Europe. Neurologists should perform bedside cognitive testing. More extensive neuropsychological testing should be primarily dedicated for mild to moderate forms of the disease, and is ideally performed by a neuropsychologist.

For neurologists, a short cognitive assessment should include a global measure, such as the MMSE, and in addition more detailed testing of the main cognitive domains. These should include: (1) word list recall; (2) temporo-spatial orientation; (3) naming; (4) drawing (the plan of the room, a cube or a clock); (5) uni- and bimanual postures execution; (6) similarities and verbal fluency.

Assessment of behavioral disorders is essential for the diagnosis and management of dementia.

The assessment should be based on caregiver interview or questionnaire using measures which investigate several behavioral domains such as the Behave-AD (Reisberg *et al*, 1987), the Neuropsychiatric Inventory (Cummings *et al*, 1994) or, for FTD, the Lund and Manchester criteria (Neary *et al*, 1998).

Assessment of activities of daily living should be included in the diagnostic evaluation and management of dementia.

Neuroimaging should be performed once in all cases of dementia referred to a neurologist. Non-contrast CT will suffice, but if available MRI is preferred and may be used to show specific abnormalities.

Functional imaging should not be used routinely, but may be of help where there is clinical suspicion of degenerative disorders and structural imaging is normal.

Laboratory screening should be included as a part of the general screening of a patient presenting with cognitive disturbances.

The following blood tests are generally proposed for all patients: blood sedimentation rate; complete blood cell count; electrolytes; glucose; renal and liver function tests; thyroid-stimulating hormone. Serological tests for the detection of Borrelia, syphilis and HIV, serum lipids, and vitamin B12 are optional. More extensive tests will often be required in individual cases.

Electrocardiography (ECG) is recommended in all patients aged above 50 years for screening purposes, in patients with cardiac symptoms or cerebrovascular lesions, and for monitoring possible side-effects in patients receiving drug therapy (e.g. acetylcholinesterase inhibitors). X-ray of chest is indicated if relevant to the symptoms.

CSF analysis (with routine cell count, protein, glucose,

and protein electrophoresis) is optional and recommended in patients with a clinical suspicion of certain diseases and in patients with atypical clinical presentations.

Electrophysiologic examination is not recommended as a routine study.

Brain biopsy is recommended in very carefully selected cases only.

It is essential to obtain consent from the patient and/or family carer and to provide counselling as identification of the mutation has clear implications for other family members.

Post mortem diagnosis of the cause of a familial degenerative dementia is critically important in future counselling for the family and should be discussed.

At present there is no clear benefit in apolipoprotein E genotyping to assist with diagnosis (Anonymous, 1995; McKeith and Morris, 1996).

Presymptomatic testing is available where there is a clear family history and where there is a known mutation in an affected individual to ensure that a negative result is clinically significant. It is recommended that the Huntington's disease protocol (Harper *et al*, 1990) is followed.

Apolipoprotein E genotyping for risk assessment is not recommended (Anonymous, 1995; McKeith and Morris, 1996).

A therapeutic trial with an AChE-I may be considered in patients with mild to moderate AD (MMSE 10-26).

If a trial is given, there should be a caregiver who can assist in administering the treatment. Treatment effects and side effects should be monitored periodically and discontinuation of treatment be considered when there are no signs of benefit.

Data are still being gathered on long-term benefits, activities of daily living, and health economics. Until these data are available, decisions on a trial to treat should be on an individual physician basis.

Neurologists should be aware of non-cognitive symptoms in patients with dementia. Assessment and treatment of non-cognitive symptoms is best undertaken by multidisciplinary teams.

In a patient with dementia and problem behaviors or emotional symptoms it is important to consider non-pharmacological interventions as an adjunct – or substitute – to pharmaceutical treatment.

Assessment of caregivers' distress and needs and administration of intervention programs for caregivers should be an integral part of the management of patients with dementia.

All patients and or caregiver should be asked about driving.

An assessment of driving ability should be guided by current cognitive function, and by a history of accidents or errors whilst driving. Particular attention should be paid to visuospatial, visuoperceptual, praxis and frontal lobe functions together with attention.

Advice either to allow driving but to review after an interval, to cease driving, or to refer for retesting should be given. This decision must accord with the national regulations of which the neurologist must be aware.

Diagnostic evaluation and management of dementia should be included in the training of all neurologists in Europe.

Conclusions

Neurologists should play an active role in the diagnostic evaluation of patients with cognitive disturbances and have a key role in the referral to and interpretation of certain ancillary investigations (lumbar puncture, neuropsychological testing, brain imaging, brain biopsy).

For some patients the neurologist is the primary physician in charge of the treatment and care. In these circumstances the neurologist should take part in the general management and in specific psychosocial treatments and assure the organization of psychosocial interventions for patients as well as for caregivers in collaboration with the community facilities. For most patients the neurologist acts as a consultant, but should be aware of available psychosocial treatment principles and caregiver intervention programs and refer the patients to appropriate programs.

There are inadequate data on the cost-effectiveness of practice parameters for diagnostic evaluation and treatment of dementia. Therefore, the recommendations in this guideline are consensus recommendations based on individual patient management, and their practice has to be in the light of available resources.

There is a clear need to clarify the role of the neurologist. Our review of the management of dementia in European countries revealed considerable differences. In some countries neurologists have taken the lead in the management of patients with dementia, while in other countries the neurologist is rarely involved. We recommend that neurologists should have a clear role in the management of dementia in the whole of Europe. Neurologists should be involved in the diagnostic evaluation of dementia, and facilitate the development of multidisciplinary teams for diagnostic evaluation of patients with cognitive disturbances and dementia. After the diagnostic evaluation the neurologist should ensure that the management of patients with dementia includes mutlidisciplinary multi-agency collaboration.

It is essential that diagnostic evaluation and management of dementia should be included in the training of all neurologists.

Additional references

Anonymous (1995). Statement on use of apolipoprotein E testing for Alzheimer disease. American College of Medical Genetics/American Society of Human Genetics Working

Group on ApoE and Alzheimer disease. *Journal of the American Medical Association* 274:1627–9.

Cummings JL, Mega M, Gray K, Rosenberg-Thompson S, Carusi DA, Gornbein J (1994). The Neuropsychiatric Inventory. Comprehensive assessment of psychopathology in dementia. *Neurology* 44: 2308–14.

Harper PS, Morris MJ, Tyler A (1990). Genetic testing for Huntington's Disease. *BMJ* 300: 1089–90.

McKeith IG, Morris CM (1996). Apolipoprotein E genotyping in Alzheimer's disease [letter]. *Lancet* 347: 1775.

Neary D, Snowden JS, Gustafson L, Passant U, Stuss D, Black S, Freedman M, Kertesz A, Robert PH, Albert M, Boone K, Miller BL, Cummings J, Benson DF (1998). Frontotemporal lobar degeneration: a consensus on clinical diagnostic criteria. *Neurology* 51: 1546–54.

Reisberg B, Borenstein J, Salob SP, Ferris SH, Franssen E, Georgotas A (1987). Behavioural symptoms in Alzheimer's disease. Phenomenology and treatment. *Journal of Clinical Psychiatry* 48(Suppl): 9–15.

Address for correspondence
Gunhild Waldemar
Department of Neurology
Copenhagen University Hospital
Rigshospitalet, N2082
9, Blegdamsvej DK-2100
Copenhagen
Denmark

Practice Guidelines for the Clinical Assessment and Care Management of Alzheimer's Disease and Other Dementias Among Adults with Intellectual Disability

Reference   Janicki MP, Heller T, Seltzer GB, Hogg J (1996) Practice guidelines for the clinical assessment and care management of Alzheimer's disease and other dementias among adults with intellectual disability. *Journal of Intellectual Disability Research* 40: 374–82

Purpose

To develop guidelines from an international group to provide guidance for stage-related care management of Alzheimer's disease in people with learning disability. These guidelines were developed following a meeting of an international workgroup, and are called the AAMR/IASSID guidelines (the American Association on Mental Retardation and the International Association for the Scientific Study of Intellectual Disability).

Summary

Three steps are recommended in the guidelines.

Step 1 Understanding changes in normal ageing, being aware of risk factors and recognizing changes indicating the onset of dementia

It is noted that it is very common for people over the age of 40 with Down's syndrome to develop Alzheimer's disease, and it is recommended that periodic screening takes place. Changes that may be early indicators of the onset of dementia include unexpected changes in routine behaviors, a decrement in functional abilities such as cooking, dressing and washing, memory losses or difficulty in learning new activities, changes in affect or attitude or demeanor, loss of job or social skills, withdrawal from pleasurable activities, night-time awakenings and other altered time difficulties, increases or decreases in rigid behavioral pattern, and the onset of seizures. Referral for a diagnostic workup to exclude other causes of dementia is recommended. It is also recommended that periodically an applied screening instrument should be used to establish a behavioral baseline and to obtain longitudinal measures that indicate change. However, no suggestion is made as to what such a screening test might be.

Step 2 Conducting assessments and evaluations

It is noted that, when there is a suspicion of dementia, referral for a thorough evaluation should be carried out, and this process should include: (a) gathering information on behavior to further confirm and notice changes, preferably from multiple informants such as staff or carers; (b) continuing to monitor behavior/functioning for presentation to clinicians; and (c) making a referral for a diagnostic workup for a differential diagnosis.

Step 3 Instituting medical and care management

The importance of medical management is emphasized (treatment of associated medical conditions, associated mental disorders, attention to sensory deficits which may exacerbate problems, and drug treatment (where appropriate) of behavioral disturbances). Care management includes documenting and carrying out a treatment strategy along the general principles of care management, i.e. helping the person preserve and maximize function by using interventions and supports that are appropriate to the stage of the disease, and conducting care planning that is multidisciplinary and involves information from multiple sources. The need for education and training and care practice policies is emphasized.

An associated document describes the epidemiology of Alzheimer's disease in mental retardation.

Conclusion

During the last decade research has made great strides toward understanding the role Alzheimer's disease plays in the lives of people with mental retardation, especially those with Down's syndrome. Yet considerably more needs to be learned:

1. Studies focusing on incidence and prevalence rates, risk factors and natural history of the disease need to be conducted and then replicated.
2. Evaluation of adults with mental retardation without Down's syndrome, a much larger group than those with Down's syndrome, should be emphasized
3. Collection of the minimum data set suggested above, by various investigators, should allow meta-analytic studies of sufficient breadth and depth to be conducted to develop and validate hypotheses regarding the variables of interest specified above
4. Studies including national and international collaboration should be undertaken to utilize shared data and knowledge
5. Efforts should be made by researchers and clinicians alike to interest funding agencies to support research in these areas.

Address for correspondence

Matthew P Janicki PhD
NYS, OMRDD
44 Holland Avenue
Albany, NY 12229
USA

Clinical Diagnosis of Alzheimer's Disease: Report of the NINCDS–ADRDA Work Group under the Auspices of Department of Health and Human Services Task Force on Alzheimer's Disease

Reference   McKhann G, Drachman D, Folstein M, Katzman R, Price D, Stadlan EM (1984) Clinical diagnosis of Alzheimer's disease: report of the NINCDS-ADRDA Work Group under the auspices of Department of Health and Human Services Task Force on Alzheimer's Disease. *Neurology* 34: 939–44

Purpose

These are the clinical diagnostic criteria which are regarded as the gold standard for the diagnosis of Alzheimer's disease – intended to serve as a guide for the diagnosis of probable/possible indefinite Alzheimer's disease.

Summary

See Tables.

Address for correspondence

Dr Stadlan
7550 Wisconsin Avenue
Federal Building
Room 700
Bethesda, MD 20205
USA

Neuropsychological evaluation

The major cognitive processes that are impaired in Alzheimer's disease, with examples of the kinds of tests used to assess these functions include:

orientation to place and time, graded by a test such as the Mini-Mental State Examination

memory evaluated by tests such as a free-recall test of concrete nouns, a 3–4 paired-associate learning test (verbal and non-verbal) by use of a recognition paradigm, the Recognition Span Test and the Brown–Peterson Distractor Test (stopping the task when the patient fails or begins to produce the distractor instead of the stimulus trigrams)

language skills tested by examination of verbal fluency of the semantic or category type, with the examiner writing responses, and by other tests such as the Boston Naming Test (preferably one of the abbreviated forms), the Boston Diagnostic Aphasia Examination, the Western Aphasia Test and the Token Test with Reporter's Test

praxis evaluated by tests such as those in which the patient copies a drawing (cube, daisy, clock or house) or performs the block design sub-test of the Wechsler Adult Intelligence Scale

attention monitored by tests such as a reaction-time task or by the Continuous-Performance Test

visual perception studied by use of a variety of tasks such as the Gollin Incomplete-Pictures Test and the Hooper Test

problem-solving skills determined by tests such as the Wisconsin Card Sorting Test or the Poisoned Food Problem Task of Arenberg and

social function, activities of daily living and instrumental activity of daily living, assessed by methods similar to those described in the Philadelphia Geriatrics Center Forms.

NINCDS-ADRDA, National Institute of Neurological and Communicative Disorders and Stroke and the Alzheimer's Disease and Related Disorders Association

Diagnostic criteria

I.   The criteria for the clinical diagnosis of PROBABLE Alzheimer's disease include:

dementia established by clinical examination and documented by the Mini-Mental Test, Blessed Dementia Scale or some similar examination and confirmed by neuropsychological tests

deficits in two or more areas of cognitive functions

no disturbance of consciousness

onset between ages 40 and 90, most often after age 65, and

absence of systemic disorders or other brain diseases that in and of themselves could account for the progressive deficits in memory and cognition.

II. The diagnosis of PROBABLE Alzheimer's disease is supported by:

progressive deterioration of specific cognitive functions such as language (aphasia), motor skills (apraxia) and perception (agnosia):

impaired activities of daily living and altered patterns of behavior

family history of similar disorders, particularly if confirmed neuropathologically, and

laboratory results of:

normal lumbar puncture as evaluated by standard techniques

normal pattern or non-specific changes in EEG, such as increased slow-wave activity and

evidence of cerebral atrophy on CT with progression documented by serial observation.

III. Other clinical features consistent with the diagnosis of PROBABLE Alzheimer's disease after exclusion of causes of dementia other than Alzheimer's disease include:

plateaus in the course of progression of the illness

associated symptoms of depression, insomnia, incontinence, delusions, illusions, hallucinations, catastrophic verbal, emotional or physical outbursts, sexual disorders and weight loss; other neurologic abnormalities in some patients, especially with more advanced disease and including motor signs such as increased muscle tone, myoclonus or gait disorder.

Seizures in advance disease, and

CT normal for age.

IV. Features that make the diagnosis of PROBABLE Alzheimer's disease uncertain or unlikely include:

sudden, apoplectic onset

focal neurologic findings such as hemiparesis, sensory loss, visual field deficits and incoordination early in the course of the illness

seizures or gait disturbances at the onset or very early in the course of the illness.

V.   Clinical diagnosis of POSSIBLE Alzheimer's disease:

may be made on the basis of the dementia syndrome in the absence of other neurologic, psychiatric or systemic disorders sufficient to cause dementia and in the presence of variations in the onset, in the presentation, or in the clinical course

may be made in the presence of a second systemic or brain disorder sufficient to produce dementia, which is not considered to be the cause of the dementia; and

should be used in research studies when a single, gradually progressive severe cognitive deficit is identified in the absence of other identifiable cause.

VI. Criteria for diagnosis of DEFINITE Alzheimer's disease are:

the clinical criteria for probable Alzheimer's disease and

histopathologic evidence obtained from a biopsy or autopsy.

VII. Classification of Alzheimer's disease for research purposes should specify features that may differentiate subtypes of the disorder, such as:

familial occurrence

onset before age of 65

presence of trisomy-21, and

coexistence of other relevant conditions such as Parkinson's disease.

Consensus Recommendations for the Postmortem Diagnosis of Alzheimer's Disease

Reference (1997) Consensus recommendations for the postmortem diagnosis of Alzheimer's disease. *Neurobiology of Aging* 18: S1–S2

Purpose

To improve the neuropathological criteria for the post mortem diagnosis of Alzheimer's disease.

Summary

The recommendations followed a 2-day workshop sponsored by the National Institute on Aging and the Ronald and Nancy Reagan Institute of the Alzheimer's Association to reassess the original criteria for the post mortem diagnosis of Alzheimer's disease (Khachaturian Z (1985) Diagnosis of Alzheimer's disease. *Archives of Neurology* 42: 1097–106).

The recommendations were summarized under five headings:

1. Guiding principles for the diagnosis of Alzheimer's disease
2. Neuropathological assessment
3. Specific recommendations
4. Assessment of major coexisting lesions in addition to Alzheimer's disease lesions in the post mortem brain
5. Recommendations for strategies to improve the post mortem diagnosis of Alzheimer's disease.

The CERAD protocol (Mirra *et al*, 1991) was endorsed.

Additional reference

Mirra SS, Heyman A, McKeel D *et al* (1991) The consortium to establish a registry for Alzheimer's disease (CERAD). II Standardization of the neuropathological assessment of Alzheimer's disease. *Neurology* 41: 479–86

Address for correspondence

Dr Johan Q Trojanowski
Working Group Chair
Dept of Pathology and Laboratory Medicine
University of Pennsylvania School of Medicine
HUP Maloney Bldg
Room A009
Philadelphia, PA 19104-4283
USA

Criteria for the Diagnosis of Ischemic Vascular Dementia Proposed by the State of California Alzheimer's Disease Diagnostic and Treatment Centers

Reference   Chui HC, Victoroff JI, Margolin D, Jagust W, Shankle R, Katzman R (1992) Criteria for the diagnosis of ischemic vascular dementia proposed by the State of California Alzheimer's Disease Diagnostic and Treatment Centers. *Neurology* 42: 473–80

Purpose

To present standardized diagnostic criteria for vascular dementia following the model of the NINCDS-ADRDA criteria for Alzheimer's disease.

Summary

The criteria broaden the conceptualization of vascular dementia, and include the results from neuroimaging studies and emphasize the importance of pathological confirmation of the diagnosis (see Table). 'Possible' and 'mixed' categories, where both Alzheimer's disease and ischaemic vascular dementia exist, are proposed (see Table).

Address for correspondence

Dr Helena Chang Chui
Geriatric Neurobehavior and Alzheimer Center
Rancho Los Amigos Medical Center
12838 Erickson Street
Downey, CA 50242
USA

Criteria for the diagnosis of ischemia vascular dementia (IVD)

I. Dementia

Dementia is a deterioration from a known or estimated prior level of intellectual function sufficient to interfere broadly with the conduct of the patient's customary affairs of life, which is not isolated to a single narrow category of intellectual performance, and which is independent of level of consciousness.

This deterioration should be supported by historical evidence and documented by either bedside mental status testing or ideally by more detailed neuropsychological examination, using tests that are quantifiable, reproducible, and for which normative data are available.

II. Probable IVD

A. The criteria for the clinical diagnosis of PROBABLE IVD include ALL of the following:
1. Dementia
2. Evidence of two or more ischemic strokes by history, neurologic signs, and/or neuroimaging studies (CT or T_1-weighted MRI)
   or
   occurrence of a single stroke with a clearly documented temporal relationship to the onset of dementia
3. Evidence of at least one infarct outside the cerebellum by CT or T_1-weighted MRI.

B. The diagnosis of PROBABLE IVD is supported by:
1. Evidence of multiple infarcts in brain regions known to affect cognition
2. A history of multiple transient ischemic attacks
3. History of vascular risk factors (e.g. hypertension, heart disease, diabetes mellitus)
4. Elevated Hachinski Ischemia Scale (original or modified version).

C. Clinical features that are thought to be associated with IVD, but await further research, include:
1. Relatively early appearance of gait disturbance and urinary incontinence
2. Periventricular and deep white matter changes on T_2-weighted MRI that are excessive for age
3. Focal changes in electrophysiologic studies (e.g. EEG, evoked studies (e.g. SPECT, PET, NMR spectroscopy).

D. Other clinical features that do not constitute strong evidence either for or against a diagnosis of PROBABLE IVD include:
1. Periods of slowly progressive symptoms
2. Illusions, psychosis, hallucinations, delusions
3. Seizures.

E. Clinical features that cast doubt on a diagnosis of PROBABLE IVD include:
1. Transcortical sensory aphasia in the absence of corresponding focal lesions on neuroimaging studies
2. Absence of central neurologic symptoms/signs, other than cognitive disturbance.

III. Possible IVD

A clinical diagnosis of POSSIBLE IVD may be made when there is
1. Dementia
   and one or more of the following:
2a. A history or evidence of a single stroke (but not multiple strokes) without a clearly documented temporal relationship to the onset of dementia
   or
2b. Binswanger's syndrome (without multiple strokes) that includes all of the following:
   i. Early-onset urinary incontinence not explained by urologic disease, or gait disturbance (e.g. parkinsonian, magnetic, apraxic, or 'senile' gait) not explained by peripheral cause
   ii. Vascular risk factors, and
   iii. Extensive white matter changes on neuroimaging.

IV. Definite IVD

A diagnosis of DEFINITE IVD requires histopathologic examination of the brain, as well as:
1. Clinical evidence of dementia
2. Pathologic confirmation of multiple infarcts, some outside of the cerebellum.

Note: If there is evidence of Alzheimer's disease or some other pathologic disorder that is thought to have contributed to the dementia, a diagnosis of MIXED dementia should be made.

V. Mixed dementia

A diagnosis of MIXED dementia should be made in the presence of one or more other systemic or brain disorders that are thought to be causally related to the dementia. The degree of confidence in the diagnosis of IVD should be specified as possible, probable, or definite, and the other disorder(s) contributing to the dementia should be listed. For example: mixed dementia due to probable IVD and possible Alzheimer's disease or mixed dementia due to definite IVD and hypothyroidism.

VI. Research classification

Classification of IVD for RESEARCH purposes should specify features of the infarcts that may differentiate subtypes of the disorder, such as

Location:	cortical, white matter, periventricular, basal ganglia, thalamus
Size:	volume
Distribution:	large, small, or microvessel
Severity:	chronic ischemia versus infarction
Etiology:	embolism, atherosclerosis, arteriosclerosis, cerebral amyloid angiopathy, hypoperfusion.

Vascular Dementia: Diagnostic Criteria for Research Studies

Reference   Roman GC, Tatemichi TK, Erkinjuntti T *et al* (1993) Vascular dementia: diagnostic criteria for research studies. Report of the NINDS–AIREN international Workshop (National Institute of Neurological Disorders and Stroke – Association Internationale pour la Recherche et l'Enseignement en Neurosciences). *Neurology* 43: 250–60

Purpose

To provide diagnostic criteria for research into vascular dementia along the lines of the celebrated NINCDS–ADRDA criteria for Alzheimer's disease.

Summary

VaD is a complex disorder characterized by cognitive impairment resulting from ischemic or hemorrhagic stroke or from ischemic-hypoxic brain lesions. The clinical criteria for the diagnosis of probable, possible and definite vascular dementia are summarized here.

I. The criteria for the clinical diagnosis of *probable* vascular dementia include *all* of the following:

1. *Dementia* defined by cognitive decline from a previously higher level of functioning and manifested by impairment of memory and of two or more cognitive domains (orientation, attention, language, visuospatial functions, executive functions, motor control and praxis), preferably established by clinical examination and documented by neuropsychological testing; deficits should be severe enough to interfere with activities of daily living not due to physical effects of stroke alone. *Exclusion criteria* include cases with disturbance of consciousness, delirium, psychosis, severe aphasia or major sensorimotor impairment precluding neuropsychological testing. Also excluded are systemic disorders or other brain diseases (such as AD) that of themselves could account for deficits in memory and cognition.
2. *Cerebrovascular disease*, defined by the presence of focal signs on neurological examination, such as hemiparesis, lower facial weakness, Babinski sign, sensory deficit, hemianopia, and dysarthria consistent with stroke (with or without history of stroke) and evidence of relevant CVD by brain imaging (CT or MRI) including *multiple large-vessel infarcts* or a *single strategically placed infarct* (gangular gyrus, thalamus, basal forebrain, or PCA or ACA territories), as well as *multiple basal ganglia* and *white matter lacunes* or *extensive periventricular white matter lesions*, or combinations thereof.
3. *A relationship between the above two disorders* manifested or inferred by the presence of one or more of the following: (a) onset of dementia within 3 months following a recognized stroke; (b) abrupt deterioration in cognitive functions, or fluctuating, stepwise progression of cognitive deficits.

II. Clinical features consistent with the diagnosis of *probably* vascular dementia include the following:

1. Early presence of a gait disturbance (small-step gait or marche à petit pas, or magnetic apraxic-ataxic or Parkinsonian gait).
2. History of unsteadiness and frequent, unprovoked falls.
3. Early urinary frequency, urgency and other urinary symptoms not explained by urologic disease.
4. Pseudobulbar palsy.
5. Personality and mood changes, abulia, depression, emotional incontinence, or other subcortical deficits including psychomotor retardation and abnormal executive function.

III. Features that make the diagnosis of vascular dementia uncertain or unlikely include:

1. Early onset of memory deficit and progressive worsening of memory and other cognitive functions such as language (transcortical sensory aphasia), motor skills (apraxia), and perception (agnosia) in the absence of corresponding focal lesions on brain imaging.
2. Absence of focal neurologic signs, other than cognitive disturbance.
3. Absence of cerebrovascular lesions on brain CT or MRI.

IV. Clinical diagnosis of *possible* vascular dementia may be made in the presence of dementia with focal neurological signs in patients in whom brain imaging studies to confirm definite CVD are missing; or in the absence of clear temporal relationship between dementia and stroke; or in patients with subtle onset and variable course (plateau or improvement) of cognitive deficits and evidence of relevant CVD.

V. Criteria for diagnosis of *definite* vascular dementia are:

1. Clinical criteria for *probably* vascular dementia.
2. Histopathologic evidence of CVD obtained from biopsy or autopsy.
3. Absence of neurofibrillary tangles and neuritic plaques exceeding those expected for age.
4. Absence of other clinical or pathologic disorder capable of producing dementia.

VI. Classification of vascular dementia for research purposes may be made on the basis of clinical, radiologic and neuropathologic features, for sub-categories or defined conditions such as cortical vascular dementia, subcortical vascular dementia, BD and thalmic dementia.

The term 'AD *with* CVD' should be reserved to classify patients fulfilling the clinical criteria for possible AD and who also present clinical or brain imaging evidence of relevant CVD. Traditionally, these patients have been included with VaD in epidemiologic studies. The term 'mixed dementia', used hitherto, should be avoided.

Topography

Radiologic lesions associated with dementia include ANY of the following or combinations thereof:

1. Large-vessel strokes in the following territories:
   - bilateral anterior cerebral artery
   - posterior cerebral artery, including paramedian thalamic infarctions, inferior medial temporal lobe lesions
   - association areas – parietotemporal, temporo-occipital territories (including angular gyrus)
   - watershed carotid territories – superior frontal, parietal regions.

2. Small vessel disease:
   - basal ganglia and frontal white matter lacunes
   - extensive periventricular white matter lacunes
   - bilateral thalamic lesions.

Severity

In addition to the above, relevant radiologic lesions associated with dementia include:

1. Large-vessel lesions of the dominant hemisphere
2. Bilateral large-vessel hemispheric strokes
3. Leukoencephalopathy involving at least $\frac{1}{4}$ of the total white matter.

Although volume of lesion is weakly related to dementia, an additive effect may be present. White matter changes observed only on T_2MRI but not on T_1. MRI or CT may not be significant. Absence of vascular lesions on brain CT/MRI *rules out* probable vascular dementia.

Address for correspondence

Dr Gustavo C Roman
Neuroepidemiology Branch
NINDS, Federal Building Room 714
Bethesda, MD 20892
USA

Consensus Guidelines for the Clinical and Pathologic Diagnosis of Dementia with Lewy Bodies (DLB): Report of the Consortium on DLB International Workshop

Reference   McKeith IG, Galasko D, Kosaka K *et al* (1996) Consensus guidelines for the clinical and pathologic diagnosis of dementia with Lewy bodies (DLB): report of the consortium on DLB international workshop. *Neurology* 47: 1113–24

Purpose

To establish operational diagnostic criteria for dementia of the Lewy body type, bringing together proponents of the previous diagnostic criteria from workers in Nottingham and Newcastle. Resulting from a consensus meeting.

Additional references

Byrne EJ, Lennox G, Godwin Austen RB *et al* (Nottingham Group for the Study of Neurodegenerative Disorders) (1991) Diagnostic criteria for dementia associated with cortical Lewy bodies. *Dementia* 2: 283–4.

McKeith I, Perry RH, Fairbairn AF, Jabeen S, Perry EK (1992) Operational criteria for senile dementia of Lewy body type (SDLT) *Psychological Medicine* 22: 911–22.

McKeith IG, Perry EK, Perry RH (1999) Report of the second dementia with Lewy body International Workshop: diagnosis and treatment. Consortium on Dementia with Lewy Bodies *Neurology* 53: 902–5.

Address for correspondence

Professor Ian McKeith
Dept of Old Age Psychiatry
Institute for the Health of the Elderly
Newcastle General Hospital
Westgate Road
Newcastle upon Tyne NE4 6BE
UK

email: i.g.mckeith@ncl.ac.uk

Consensus criteria for the clinical diagnosis of probable and possible DLB

1. The central feature required for a diagnosis of DLB is progressive cognitive decline of sufficient magnitude to interfere with normal social or occupational function. Prominent or persistent memory impairment may not necessarily occur in the early stages but is usually evident with progression. Deficits on tests of attention and of frontal-subcortical skills and visuospatial ability may be especially prominent.
2. Two of the following core features are essential for a diagnosis of probable DLB, and one is essential for possible DLB:
   (a) Fluctuating cognition with pronounced variations in attention and alertness.
   (b) Recurrent visual hallucinations that are typically well formed and detailed.
   (c) Spontaneous motor features of parkinsonism.
3. Features supportive of the diagnosis are
   (a) Repeated falls
   (b) Syncope
   (c) Transient loss of consciousness
   (d) Neuroleptic sensitivity
   (e) Systematized delusions
   (f) Hallucinations in other modalities.
4. A diagnosis of DLB is less likely in the presence of
   (a) Stroke disease, evident as focal neurologic signs or on brain imaging.
   (b) Evidence on physical examination and investigation of any physical illness or other brain disorder sufficient to account for the clinical picture.

Clinical and Neuropathological Criteria for Frontotemporal Dementia

Reference   **The Lund and Manchester Groups (1994) Clinical and neuropathological criteria for frontotemporal dementia.** *Journal of Neurology, Neurosurgery and Psychiatry* **57: 416–18**

Purpose

To define clinical and pathological criteria for frontotemporal dementia.

Summary

Clinical diagnostic features of frontotemporal dementia

Core diagnostic features include:

1. *Behavioural disorder*
   - insidious onset and slow progression
   - early loss of personal awareness (neglect of personal hygiene and grooming)
   - early loss of social awareness (lack of social tact, misdemeanours such as shoplifting)
   - early signs of disinhibition (such as unrestrained sexuality, violent behaviour, inappropriate jocularity, restless pacing)
   - mental rigidity and inflexibility
   - hyperorality (oral/dietary changes, food fads, excessive smoking and alcohol consumption, oral exploration of objects)
   - stereotyped and preservative behaviour (wandering, mannerisms such as clapping, singing, dancing, ritualistic preoccupations such as hoarding, toileting and dressing)
   - utilization behaviour (unrestrained exploration of objects in the environment)
   - distractibility, impulsivity and impersistence
   - early loss of insight into the fact that the altered condition is due to a pathological change of own mental state.
2. *Affective symptoms*
   - depression, anxiety, excessive sentimentality, suicidal and fixed ideation, delusion (early and evanescent)
   - hypochondriasis, bizarre somatic preoccupation (early evanescent)
   - emotional unconcern (emotional indifference and remoteness, lack of empathy and sympathy, apathy)
   - amimia (inertia, aspontaneity).
3. *Speech disorder*
   - progressive reduction of speech (aspontaneity and economy of utterance)
   - stereotypy of speech (repetition of limited repertoire of words, phrases or themes)
   - Echolalia and preservation
   - Late mutism.
4. *Spatial orientation and praxis preserved* (intact abilities to negotiate the environment)
5. *Physical signs*
   - early primitive reflexes
   - early incontinence
   - late akinesia, rigidity, tremor
   - low and labile blood pressure.
6. *Investigations*
   - normal EEG despite clinically evident dementia
   - brain imaging (structural or functional, or both); predominant frontal or anterior temporal abnormality, or both
   - neuropsychology (profound failure on 'frontal lobe' tests in the absence of severe amnesia, aphasia or perceptual spatial disorder).

Supportive diagnostic features include:

1. Onset before 65
2. Positive family history of similar disorder in a first degree relative
3. Bulbar palsy, muscular weakness and wasting, fasciculations (motor neuron disease).

Diagnostic exclusion features include:

1. Abrupt onset with ictal events
2. Head trauma related to onset
3. Early severe amnesia
4. Early spatial disorientation, lost in surroundings, defective localization of objects
5. Early severe apraxia
6. Logoclonic speech with rapid loss of train of thought
7. Myoclonus
8. Cortical bulbar and spinal deficits
9. Cerebellar ataxia
10. Choreo-athetosis
11. Early, severe, pathological EEG
12. Brain imaging (predominant post-central structural or functional deficit, multifocal cerebral lesions on CT or MRI)
13. Laboratory tests indicating brain involvement or inflammatory disorder (such as multiple sclerosis, syphilis, AIDS and herpes simplex encephalitis).

Relative diagnostic exclusion features include:

1. Typical history of chronic alcoholism
2. Sustained hypertension
3. History of vascular disease (such as angina, claudication).

Neuropathological criteria are described for frontal lobe degeneration: gross changes (including slight symmetrical convolutional atrophy in frontal and anterior temporal lobe with widened ventricles frontally); distribution of microscopic changes (changes seen in the frontal convexity and in the anterior third of the temporal cortex with sparing of the superior temporal gyrus and usually the parietal lobe); and microscopic characteristics (microvacuolation and astrocytic gliosis in the grey matter with loss of neurons in laminae II and III and the absence of Pick bodies, astrocytic gliosis with ischaemic white matter changes in the white matter).

Pick type: frontotemporal dementia – gross changes (the same localization as in frontal lobe degeneration but usually more severe and circumscribed); microscopic changes (of the same distribution as in frontotemporal dementia); microscopic changes in the grey and white matter (intense involvement of all cortical layers with inflated neurones and Pick bodies and more intense white matter involvement).

Motor neurone disease type: gross changes (as in frontal lobe degeneration); microscopic changes (the same as for frontal lobe degeneration but with additional spinal motor neurone degeneration affecting cervical and thoracic levels

with inclusion bodies in layer II of the frontal and temporal cortex which are ubiquiton positive); the presence of senile plaques, amyloid deposits, amyloid angiopathy and tangles more than would be expected for age; and the presence of prion protein antibodies.

Additional reference

Neary D, Snowden JS, Gustafson L *et al* (1998) Frontotemporal lobar degeneration. A consensus on clinical diagnostic criteria. *Neurology* 51: 1546–54.

Neary provided an overview of the criteria emphasizing that there is no indication of the relative importance of behavioural features and whether a specified number of features are needed to be present. Also, it was not stated explicitly whether additional investigations such as EEG, neuropsychological tests or brain imaging are included and no operational definitions are provided of the descriptive terms. Finally, the behavioural disorder of frontotemporal dementia is only one of the potential clinical manifestations of the disorder.

Address for correspondence

Professor David Neary
Dept of Neurology
Manchester Royal Infirmary
Manchester M13 9WL
UK

Guidance on the Use of Donepezil, Rivastigmine and Galantamine for the Treatment of Alzheimer's Disease

Reference: National Institute for Clinical Excellence (2001). Technology Appraisal Guidance No. 19

Purpose

Appraisal of the available evidence on cholinesterase inhibitors in order to produce national guidance for clinicians and health commissioners. Health professionals are expected to take it fully into account when exercising their clinical judgement about the use of these drugs. The guidance does not, however, override the clinician's individual responsiblity to make appropriate decisions in the circumstances of the individual patient.

Summary

1. Guidance

1.1   The three drugs donepezil, rivastigmine and galantamine should be made available in the NHS as one component of the management of those people with mild and moderate Alzheimer's disease (AD) whose mini mental state examination (MMSE) score is above 12 points under the following conditions:

1.1.1 Diagnosis that the form of dementia is AD must be made in a specialist clinic according to standard diagnostic criteria.

1.1.2 Assessment in a specialist clinic, including tests of cognitive, global and behavioural functioning and of activities of daily living, should be made before the drug is prescribed.

1.1.3 Clinicians should also exercise judgement about the likelihood of compliance; in general, a carer or care-worker who is in sufficient contact with the patient to ensure compliance should be a minimum requirement.

1.1.4 Only specialists (including Old Age Psychiatrists, Neurologists, and Care of the Elderly Physicians) should initiate treatment. Carers' views of the patient's condition at baseline and follow-up should be sought. If General Practitioners are to take over prescribing, it is recommended that they should do so under an agreed shared care protocol with clear treatment end points.

1.1.5 A further assessment should be made, usually two to four months after reaching maintenance dose of the drug. Following this assessment the drug should be continued only when there has been an improvement or no deterioration in MMSE score, together with evidence of global improvement on the basis of behavioural and/or functional assessment.

1.1.6 Patients who continue on the drug should be reviewed by MMSE score and global, functional and behavioural assessment every 6 months. The drug should normally only be continued while their MMSE score remains above 12 points, and their global, functional and behavioural condition remains at a level where the drug is considered to be having a worthwhile effect. When the MMSE score falls below 12 points, patients should not normally be prescribed any of these three drugs. Any review involving MMSE assessment should be undertaken by an appropriate specialist team, unless there are locally-agreed protocols for shared care.

1.2   The benefits of these three drugs for patients with other forms of dementia (e.g. Dementia with Lewy Bodies) has not been assessed in this guidance.

Other sections of the guidance are as follows:

2. Clinical Need and Practice
3. The Technology
4. Evidence
5. Implications for the NHS

The total drug cost to the UK National Health Service is estimated at around £42 million per annum once a steady state of prescribing is reached. Additional costs will arise from the need for more specialist assessment, investigation and monitoring. There may be savings if the entry to nursing and residential home care is delayed, but the extent of this is not clear.

6. Further research

Is needed to identify:

– whether these drugs are of similar effectiveness
– whether their effect establishes itself immediately and then declines, or whether they have a cumulative effect over time and influence the course of the disease
– the extent of adverse effects over time, particularly in relation to dosage
– the place of these drugs in the treatment of severe dementia
– the place of these drugs in the management of non-cognitive symptoms and behavioural disturbance in dementia
– whether these drugs are of benefit in other forms of dementia

–   whether patients who come off the drug maintain benefits, decline to the level they would have been without the drug, or decline even further
–   the effects of the drugs on the delay in institutionalisation, and therefore their overall cost-effectiveness.

7. Implementation
8. Clinical audit advice
9. Review of guidance – December 2003

Address for correspondence

National Institute for Clinical Excellence

11 Strand

London

WC2N 5HR

UK

www.nice.org.uk

The Use of Donepezil for Alzheimer's Disease

Reference   Standard Medical Advisory Committee (1998) UK Dept of Health

Purpose

To provide guidance for clinicians for the use of donepezil in Alzheimer's disease (although specific for donepezil, the guideline should be used for all of the anticholinesterase drugs).

Summary

The Standing Medical Advisory Committee (SMAC) recommends that treatment with donepezil should be initiated and supervised only by a specialist experienced in the management of dementia. Benefit should be assessed at 12 weeks. Treatment should continue only for those patients with evidence of benefit.

Background

1. In spring 1997 SMAC endorsed an interim statement by the Royal College of Psychiatrists on new anti-dementia medicines. Since then several further assessments of donepezil (Aricept, Eisai/Pfizer), which is licensed for the treatment of mild to moderate Alzheimer's disease, have been produced and the results of two clinical trials have been published. Ministers have asked SMAC to prepare brief guidance to clinicians.

2. Donepezil is one of a new group of acetylcholinesterase inhibitors which has been licensed in the UK for use with people with mild to moderate Alzheimer's disease. The drug is marketed as having an effect on the manifestations of the disease – it has no apparent effect on the underlying disease process. The product licence states that "Diagnosis and treatment must be under supervision of a clinician experienced in Alzheimer's dementia". The cost of donepezil is approximately £1,000 per patient per year.

General principles

3. SMAC considers that it is important for clinicians not only to assess the benefits to individual patients, but also to be sensitive to the needs of the population as a whole. Resources should not be diverted to treatments whose clinical benefit and cost effectiveness is not yet proven. A principal objective should be the avoidance of wasteful prescribing, with medicines targeted on those patients who will benefit most.

4. In order to make an authoritative statement on the use by clinicians of any drug or treatment, SMAC would expect robust published evidence to demonstrate significant clinical benefit and would also expect to see (in confidence) all papers that have been peer reviewed and accepted for publication.

Assessment and effectiveness of donepezil

5. There are currently few published data from primary research on donepezil. The main papers relevant to anti-dementia drugs that were considered by SMAC are listed [in this report]. From the short-term studies so far available, there is evidence that donepezil produces improvement in a minority of patients with mild to moderate Alzheimer's disease (defined in the published studies as those with a Mini-Mental State Examination of between 10 and 26). There is no evidence to date that donepezil has any effect on the non-cognitive manifestations of Alzheimer's disease. The available evidence is not sufficient to give a clear verdict on the cost-effectiveness of donepezil.

Assessment and diagnosis-eligibility criteria

6. Where physicians consider that prescription of the drug is justifiable, they should ensure that treatment is carefully targeted and monitored so that patients receive the most benefit from available resources. The introduction of this treatment should therefore involve accurate diagnosis and systematic monitoring. The variation in response shown to donepezil in clinical research and the absence of factors predicting benefit make pre-treatment selection difficult. Patients should be referred for specialist evaluation by a consultant in psychiatry of old age, geriatric medicine, neurology or neuropsychiatry to establish the diagnosis. Consultants should ensure that the characteristics of patients selected for treatment are essentially the same as those described in the published studies.

Prescribing

7. Only specialists should initiate the treatment. If GPs are to take over prescribing, it is recommended they should do so only under an agreed shared-care protocol with a clear end-point.

8. The patient should be reviewed early to assess compliance and tolerance. The specialist should review the patient at 12 weeks to assess benefit and review the

dose. Prescribing should continue only if, in the specialist's judgment and informed by appropriate measures of cognition and function, benefit is confirmed. For those patients who remain on the drug on a long-term basis, continued monitoring by the specialist is necessary. The specialist will need to consider carefully whether to continue the treatment when there no longer appears to be significant benefit.

9. At present too little is known about the duration of benefit. Further controlled trials are urgently needed to determine how long prescribing is justified, even in patients who benefit initially.

Address for correspondence

Mrs Bharati Trivedi
145C Skipton House
80 London Road
Elephant and Castle
London SE1 6LH
UK

Practice Guideline for the Treatment of Patients with Alzheimer's Disease and Other Dementias of Late Life

Reference   Rabins PV, Blacker D, Bland W, Bright-Long L, Cohen E, Katz I, Rovner B, Schneider L (1997) Practice guideline for the treatment of patients with Alzheimer's disease and other dementias of late life. *American Journal of Psychiatry* 154 (Suppl): 1–39

Purpose

To assist the psychiatrist in caring for a dementing patient. Much of the emphasis in the practice guideline is on the behavioral symptoms, because most of the effective treatments available for dementing disorders are in this area. The guideline was developed under the auspices of the Steering Committee on Practice Guidelines. There was initial drafting by a workgroup that included psychiatrists with clinical research expertise in dementia, a comprehensive literature review, and the production of multiple drafts with widespread review in which 10 organizations and over 48 individuals submitted comments. There was then final approval by the APA Assembly and Board of Trustees. The guideline will be revised at 3–5-year intervals.

Summary

The general treatment principles for Alzheimer's disease patients are laid out, and recommendations on specific areas of treatment are made according to three different categories.

- Category 1 – treatment is recommended with substantial clinical confidence
- Category 2 – treatment is recommended with moderate clinical confidence
- Category 3 – treatment may be recommended on the basis of individual circumstances.

The guideline provides recommendations in the following areas: psychiatric management; specific psychotherapies and other psychosocial treatments; special concerns regarding somatic treatments for elderly and demented patients; treatment of cognitive symptoms; treatment of psychosis and agitation; treatment of depression; treatment of sleep disturbances; special issues for long-term care.

1. *Psychiatric management.* The core treatment of demented patients is psychiatric management, which must be based on a solid alliance with the patient and family and thorough psychiatric, neurological and general medical evaluations of the nature and cause of the cognitive deficits and associated non-cognitive symptoms. Ongoing assessment should include periodic monitoring of the development and evolution of cognitive and non-cognitive symptoms and their response to intervention.

2. *Specific psychotherapies and other psychosocial treatments.* Few of these treatments have been subjected to double-blind randomized evaluation, but some research, along with clinical practice, supports their effectiveness. Stimulation-oriented treatments such as recreational activity, art therapy and pet therapy have moderate support from clinical trials.

3. *Special concerns regarding somatic treatments for elderly and demented patients.* Psychoactive medications are effective in the management of some symptoms associated with dementia, but they must be used with caution.

4. *Treatment of cognitive symptoms* (at the time of publication of the guideline). Two cholinesterase inhibitors are available for Alzheimer's disease; tacrine and donepezil. Both have been shown to lead to moderate improvements in cognition in a substantial minority of patients. Vitamin E may also be considered for patients with moderate Alzheimer's disease. Selegiline may be considered for patients with moderate Alzheimer's disease to prevent further decline, and may possibly be beneficial earlier or later in the course of the disease.

5. *Treatment of psychosis and agitation.* If behavioral measures are unsuccessful, the symptoms may be treated with psychotropic agents. Benzodiazepines are most useful for treating agitation with prominent anxiety. Anticonvulsants such as carbamazepine and valproate, the sedating antidepressant trazadone, the atypical anxiolytic buspirone, and possibly SSRIs may be appropriate for non-psychotic patients with behavioral disorders, especially those with mild symptoms or sensitivity to antipsychotic medications.

6. *Treatment of depression.* Patients with depression should be carefully evaluated for suicide potential. There is considerable clinical evidence supporting the use of antidepressants in patients with dementia who are depressed. SSRIs are probably the first-line treatment. Agents with significant anticholinergic effects should be avoided.

7. *Treatment of sleep disturbances.* Pharmacological intervention should be considered only when other interventions, including careful attention to sleep hygiene, have failed. Possibly effective agents include zolpidem and trazodone. Benzodiazepines and chloral

hydrate are usually not recommended for other than brief use.

8. *Special issues for long-term care.* Facilities should be structured to meet the needs of patients with dementia, including those with behavioral problems. A particular concern is the use of physical restraints and antipsychotic medications. When used appropriately, antispychotics can relieve symptoms and reduce distress for patients, and increase safety for patients, other residents and staff. However, over-use can lead to worsening of the dementia, over-sedation, falls and tardive dyskinesia. Physical restraints should be used only for patients who pose an imminent risk of harm to themselves or others. When restraints are used, the indications and alternatives should be carefully documented.

Address for correspondence

American Psychiatric Association
1400 K Street NW
Washington DC 20005
USA

Guidelines on Drug Treatments for Alzheimer's Disease

Reference   Lovestone S, Graham N, Howard R (1997) Guidelines on drug treatments for Alzheimer's disease. *The Lancet* 350: 232–3

Purpose

To suggest UK guidelines on the prescription of drugs for Alzheimer's disease.

Summary

The guidelines suggest that drugs should be prescribed only for patients with:

- McKhann criteria for probable AD
- Duration >6 months
- MMSE 10–24.

There should be a three-phase evaluation of response:

- Early (2 weeks) for side-effects
- Later (3 months) for cognitive state
- Continued 6-monthly for disease state.

Treatment should be stopped:

- Early if there is poor tolerance or compliance
- If there is continued deterioration at the pretreatment rate after 3–6 months
- After maintenance if there is accelerating deterioration
- If a drug-free period suggests the drug is no longer helping.

Address for correspondence

Professor S Lovestone
Section of Old Age Psychiatry
Institute of Psychiatry
De Crespigny Park
Denmark Hill
London SE5 8AF
UK

Initiating and Monitoring Cholinesterase Inhibitors

Reference   Swanwick GR, Lawlor BA (1999) Initiating and monitoring cholinesterase inhibitor treatment for Alzheimer's disease. *International Journal of Geriatric Psychiatry* 14: 244–8

Purpose

A model is proposed whereby specialist monitoring using formal cognitive or functional tests is neither appropriate nor necessary to determine whether an individual patient should continue or stop cholinesterase treatment for Alzheimer's disease.

Summary

The availability of cholinesterase inhibitors for the treatment of Alzheimer's disease raises a number of clinical and ethical questions. Many of the guidelines published attempting to tackle these questions lack either clinical or scientific validity. Against this background a model is proposed whereby specialist monitoring using formal cognitive or functional tests is neither appropriate or necessary to determine whether an individual patient should continue or stop treatment. Instead, the primary care physician should refer potentially suitable patients for specialist assessment to confirm the diagnosis. He/she should then initiate, monitor and discontinue treatment based on the establishment of realistic treatment goals agreed with the patient/carer at the outset. Ultimately, the decision to initiate and continue/stop treatment will be patient, family and consumer led.

Addresses for correspondence

Dr Gregory Swanwick
Consultant in Old Age Psychiatry
Tallaght Hospital
Dublin 24
Ireland

Professor B Lawlor
Mercer's Institute on Ageing
St James's Hospital
Dublin 8
Ireland

e-mail: psychel@indigo.ie

Neuroleptics in the Elderly: Guidelines for Monitoring

Reference   Sweet RA, Pollock BG (1995) Neuroleptics in the elderly: guidelines for monitoring. *Harvard Review of Psychiatry* 2: 327–35

Purpose

In the USA, the Nursing Home Reform Amendments of the Omnibus Reconciliation Act of 1987 provided guidelines for the use of neuroleptic medications in nursing-home patients. This paper reviews the existing literature to refine the recommendations for neuroleptic dosage limits, and to derive standards for the monitoring of neuroleptic-induced movement disorders in the elderly.

Summary

This is more a review of the literature than a formal guideline, but it does contain some recommendations for practice based on the available evidence. It examines two main questions – neuroleptic dosage limits, and monitoring for drug-induced movement disorders.

On drug dosage:

- for individual patients, dose should always be titrated based on a risk–benefit assessment
- caution is needed treating elderly patients with doses of conventional neuroleptics approaching 200 mg/day chlorpromazine equivalents
- many patients will benefit from substantially lower doses and thus potentially avoid exposure to dose-related side effects

- some patients, e.g. those with non-organic psychoses, may tolerate higher doses
- to exceed 200 mg/day chlorpromazine equivalents should require justification that the patient has not deteriorated due to Parkinsonism.

Monitoring for neuroleptic-induced movement disorders:

- for Parkinsonism, weekly for 3 months after initiating or increasing dose
- for akathisia, weekly for 3 months after initiating or increasing dose
- for tardive dyskinesia, monthly for 2 years, then every 6 months indefinitely
- OBRA 87 requires attempts to reduce dosage every 6 months, but reviews should probably be more frequent, based on the clinical assessment of risk and benefit for the individual patient.

Address for correspondence

Robert A Sweet, MD
Western Psychiatric Institute and Clinic
3811 O'Hara Street
Pittsburgh, PA 15213
USA

A Review and Commentary on a Sample of 15 UK Guidelines for the Drug Treatment of Alzheimer's Disease

Reference   Harvey RJ (1999) A review and commentary on a sample of 15 UK guidelines for the drug treatment of Alzheimer's disease. *International Journal of Geriatric Psychiatry* 14: 249–56

Purpose

To provide an independent review of guidelines available in the public domain for the drug treatment of Alzheimer's disease in the UK.

Summary

Fifteen sets of guidelines were obtained from a variety of sources and reviewed in a standardized way to extract the recommendations being made in the following areas: diagnosis, investigations, the evidence base of the recommendations, initiation of drug treatment; monitoring and dose adjustment; and decision-making on maintenance or discontinuation of treatment.

None of the documents fulfilled criteria for high-quality evidence-based guidelines. Substantial variability was evident in all areas of recommendation. All of the guidelines appeared to be based upon consensus opinion. Only one incorporated a statement of potential conflicts of interest affecting the working group who developed the guideline. The lack of consistency found in the guidelines would inevitably lead to inequalities in health care delivered in different areas. A national initiative is needed to encourage true evidence-based guideline development, not only on drug treatment but also on the wider issues raised such as diagnosis, investigations and the best treatment setting for delivering drug and other therapies.

Address for correspondence

Dr R Harvey
Dementia Research Group
National Hospital for Neurology and Neurosurgery
Queen Square
London WC1N 3BG
UK

r.harvey@dementia.ion.ucl.ac.uk

Drugs and Dementia: A Guide to Good Practice in the Use of Neuroleptic Drugs in Care Homes for Older People

Reference Levenson R (1998) Drugs and dementia: a guide to good practice in the use of neuroleptic drugs in care homes for older people. London: Age Concern

Purpose

This document addresses some of the concerns about the use of neuroleptic drugs in residential care homes and nursing homes. It is intended for those involved in the care of older people in care homes, as well as being of use to older people and their relatives and friends.

Summary

This consists of seven sections with four appendices. It outlines the issues and concerns about excessive prescribing of neuroleptics and the possible consequences. The need to consider alternative approaches and to monitor prescribing is also discussed. The appendices give advice as to how to get further help and how to make a complaint.

The principles of good practice are as follows:

1. The dignity and wellbeing of the older person as an individual are the primary areas of concern.
2. A holistic approach to care is essential.
3. Decisions on drug use should be seen as part of the overall plan of care for an older person in residential care.
4. Multidisciplinary and multiprofessional teamwork is necessary in order to deliver excellent care to older people in care homes.
5. Care and treatment of older people in care homes should be based on the best available evidence in the fields of health and social care.
6. Neuroleptics should only be used for older people in care homes where other ways of treating symptoms or behavioural disorders are ineffective or inappropriate, and where there are clinical indicators for the use of neuroleptics.
7. The law relating to consent should be carefully observed.
8. Clear and high-quality information on neuroleptics should be made available to older people and their relatives.

Additional references

Lester M, Warner J (1998) Antipsychotic drugs: their use and misuse. *Journal of Dementia Care* **Jan/Feb**: 25–7

McGrath A, Jackson G (1996) Survey of neuroleptic prescribing in residents of nursing homes in Glasgow. *British Medical Journal* **312**: 1667–9

Address for correspondence

Age Concern England
Astral House
1268 London Road
London SW16 4ER
UK

Guidelines for the Clinical Evaluation of Anti-Dementia Drugs

Reference   Leber P (1990) Federal Drug Administration

Purpose

The guideline is one of a series of documents published by the FDA to assist sponsors in the development of new drug products. This particular guideline, dealing exclusively with anti-dementia drugs, provides detailed information about the nature and basis of agencies' policies which may affect the scope and pace of pre-marketing development. The guidelines are intended primarily to provide advice about matters and issues relating to the planning, design, conduct and interpretation of clinical investigations, investigations that must serve as primary sources of evidence supporting claims for the safety and efficacy of new drug products. The advice offered reflects what experts working in the field believe are scientifically sound approaches to a number of issues that in the past have posed difficulties for the developer of anti-dementia drugs. Hopefully, the sponsor who reads the advice and suggestions offered will find the demanding task of commercial drug development much facilitated (although not primarily advice of practical use to old-age psychiatrists, this document provides a very important understanding of the thinking surrounding the introduction of anti-dementia drugs).

Summary

It is essentially a descriptive document under the following headings:

- Definition of dementia
- The nature of acceptable anti-dementia drug claims
- FDA regulation of clinical drug testing and overview
- The strategy and tactics of drug development (essential prerequisites of clinical drug testing, early clinical testing, the early demonstration of efficacy)
- Ultimate goal of drug developments
- Phases of drug development as described
- Design issues outlined in detail (the need for internal controls, the value of fixed treatment level design, parallel and crossover designs)
- The choice of experimental conditions (the inter-relationship between the testing and the nature of the patients studied, subject selection criteria)
- Diagnosis (stage and severity of illness)
- Dosing issues (choosing the dose and dosing regime to study, enhancing compliance)
- Efficacy assessment (prospective identification of major outcome assessment outcome variables, specific assessments required to document an anti-dementia claim, cognitive assessments and the choice of global assessment)
- Safety assessment (overall goals of phases)
- The importance of labelling
- Practical advice.

Medicinal Products in the Treatment of Alzheimer's Disease

Reference **The European Agency for the Evaluation of Medicinal Products, Human Medicines Evaluation Unit (1997). CPMP/EWP/553/95**

Introduction

The term dementia describes a syndrome characterised by dysmnesia, intellectual deterioration, changes in personality and behavioural abnormalities (DSM-III-R, DSM-IV, ICD-10). These symptoms result in social and occupational decline. The dementia syndrome can have multiple aetiologies and pathophysiologies. Thus there can probably be no single "antidementia" drug, but different drugs should be developed directed towards either symptomatic change or to modification of aetiological and pathophysiological processes.

The principles of the present guidelines are mainly applicable to Alzheimer's disease (AD), but may be adapted for use in preparing guidance for drug trials in other specific forms of dementia.

It should be recognised that the symptomatic treatment of AD is still an open research field. The development and use of relevant reliable and sensitive instruments to measure, among others, activities of daily living (ADL), instrumental activities of daily living (IADL) and behavioural symptoms is encouraged.

I DIAGNOSIS

1 Dementia

The clinical syndrome of dementia and the criteria for its severity are defined in the Diagnostic and Statistical Manual of Mental Disorders (DSM-III. Revised 1988 and DSM-IV of the American Psychiatric Association) and in ICD-10 (F00-F03) of the WHO.

According to these definitions, the diagnosis of dementia is primarily clinical. It is based on a careful history, obtained from the patient and their relatives and caregivers. The history should demonstrate a typical progressive deterioration of cognitive and non-cognitive functions and some functional and behavioural consequences of this deterioration.

At neurological and neuropsychological examination, there must be explicit impairments in memory and other cognitive domains, in the absence of developmental deficits. These impairments should not be explained by another major primary psychiatric disorder. Simple screening tests, such as the Mini Mental State Examination (MMSE) are useful to document cognitive dysfunction.

2 Severity of dementia

The DSM-IV and ICD 10 include criteria for mild, moderate and severe dementia. The severity of cognitive impairment and behavioural changes and the resulting changes in self-care and other ADL can be documented using a variety of specific and global rating instruments. The degree of severity of dementia of the included patients should be assessed and the method used should be stated.

3 The diagnosis of Alzheimer's dementia

The probability that a dementia syndrome is caused by AD is essentially based on a history of a steadily progressive course and on the absence of evidence for any other clinically diagnosable cause of the dementia. It can be further specified by using the NINCDS-ADRDA criteria (National Institute of Neurological and Communicative Disorders and Stroke; Alzheimer's Disease and Related Disorders Association). Knowledge about AD is accumulating rapidly, thus the diagnostic criteria used may need revision and updating. Patients with brain biopsy proven definite AD are seldom available. Currently the most appropriate group in whom to study the effects of drugs are patients with probable AD, according to the NINCDS-ADRDA criteria.

4 Selection criteria for Alzheimer's disease

As stated above, the diagnosis of AD consists of two steps: first, the clinical diagnosis of dementia and second, the exclusion of other causes of dementia. This relies on a careful history with a clinical neurological examination and technical and laboratory methods. As the latter are evolving rapidly, no complete list is presented here. Other causes of dementia to be excluded with pertinent method include in particular vascular dementia, infections of CNS (e.g. HIV, syphilis), Creutzfeld-Jakob disease, Huntington's disease, and Parkinson's disease. Subdural haematoma, communicating hydrocephalus, brain tumours, drug intoxication, alcohol intoxication, thyroid disease, parathyroid disease, and vitamin or other deficiencies also need to be excluded when appropriate. The following methods are strongly recommended:

- Brain imaging, such as CT or MRI to exclude major structural brain diseases. These include ischaemic infarcts, subdural haematoma, communicating hydrocephalus and brain tumours.

- The NINDS AIREN (1993) criteria to render vascular dementia unprobable.
- Blood tests to exclude infectious, endocrine, and other systemic disorders.
- History and laboratory screening to exclude drug use and abuse. Neuroleptics, hypnotics, alcohol, opioids, benzodiazepines, other sedatives and illicit drugs should be considered, as likely or contributing causes.

The inclusion criteria, exclusion criteria, examinations, methods of examination and evaluation should be carefully described and documented.

II ASSESSMENT OF THERAPEUTIC EFFICACY IN ALZHEIMER'S DISEASE

1 Criteria of efficacy

The main goals of AD treatments may be:

- Symptomatic improvement, which may be manifest in enhanced cognition, more autonomy and/or improvement in behavioural dysfunction.
- Slowing or arrest of symptom progression.
- Primary prevention of disease by intervention in key pathogenic mechanisms at a presymptomatic stage.

This guideline will concentrate on assessment of symptomatic improvement in so far as, for the time being, experience is lacking in either slowing, arresting symptom progression or in the primary prevention of disease.

Improvement of symptoms should be assessed in the following three domains:
1) cognition, as measured by objective tests (cognitive endpoint);
2) activities of daily living (functional endpoint).
3) overall clinical response, as reflected by global assessment (global endpoint).

Efficacy variables should be specified for each of the three domains. Two primary variables should be stipulated, one of which evaluates the cognitive endpoint. The other should reflect the clinical relevance of the improvement in cognition. The protocol should specify this second primary variable and to which domain (global, or preferably functional) it relates. The study should be designed to show significant differences in at least each of the two primary variables.

If this is achieved, then an assessment should be made of the overall benefit (response) in individual patients, and the effect of treatment should be illustrated in terms of the proportion of patients who achieve a meaningful benefit (response). For a claim of short term treatment, responders may be defined at 6 months as improved to a relevant prespecified degree in the cognitive endpoint and not worsened in the two other domains. Other definitions of responders are possible, but should be justified by the applicant, taking into account the clinical relevance of the outcome.

Other end-points of interest may include behavioural symptoms. For a claim in these symptoms, a specific trial should be designed with behavioural symptoms as the primary variable measured according to a specific and validated scale.

In the more advanced forms of the disease, changes in cognitive performance may be less relevant to quantify. Hence a statistically significant improvement on the functional and global endpoints may be considered as primary evidence of clinically relevant symptomatic improvement in this population.

2 Study design and methods
2.1 Run-in period

The screening and run-in period, preceding randomisation to treatment is used for wash-out of previously administered medicinal products which are incompatible with the trial, and for the qualitative and quantitative baseline assessment of patients. Patients with major short term fluctuations of their condition should be excluded. Placebo can be given during this period to assess compliance with medication.

2.2 Choice of tools

Measurement tools (cognitive, functional or global) should be externally validated, pertinent in terms of realistically reflecting symptomatic severity, sufficiently sensitive to detect modest changes related to treatment, reliable (inter-rater; test/retest reliability) and as far as possible easy to use and of short duration, allowing the possibility of easy combination with other tests. They should be calibrated in relation to various populations or sub-populations of different social, educational and cultural backgrounds in order to have validated norms available for the interpretation of the results.

They should be standardised for use in different languages and cultures. Some tools (e.g. memory tests) should be available in several equivalent forms to allow for the effect of training with repeated administration.

Applicants may need to use several instruments to assess efficacy of putative Alzheimer's drugs because:

a) there is no single test that encompasses the broad range of heterogeneous manifestations of dementia in AD;
b) there is no ideal measurement instrument at the present time. Whilst a large number of methods for evaluation of cognitive functions and behavioural changes have been suggested, none has convincingly emerged as the reference technique, satisfying the above set of requirements. Hence the choice of assessment tools should remain open, provided that the rationale for their use is presented, and justified;
c) demented patients are poor observers and reporters of their own symptoms and behaviour: self-report measures tend therefore to be less sensitive to treatment effects

than observer-related instruments. Relatives or nurses evaluations should therefore be part of the assessment, even though the risk of bias should not be underestimated.

For each domain one instrument should be specified in the protocol as primary. If this is not done, then the resulting multiplicity issues must be addressed.

It is recommended that each domain is assessed by a different investigator who should be independent of and blind to all other ratings of outcome. If side effects exist which can unblind the investigator, all outcome raters should be denied access to this information as far as possible.

The applicant will be required to justify the instruments selected with respect to their qualities.

2.2.1 Objective cognitive tests

Objective tests of cognitive function must be included in the psychometric assessment; such tests or batteries of tests must cover more than just memory as impairments in domains other than memory are mandatory for the diagnosis of AD and the assessment of its severity. Within the domain of memory, several aspects should be assessed. These are learning of new material, remote as well as recent memory, and recall and recognition memory for various modalities (including verbal and visuo-spatial). Other cognitive domains such as language, constructional ability, attention/concentration and psycho-motor speed should be assessed as well.

The Alzheimer's Disease Assessment Scale (ADAS) cognitive subscale, dealing with memory, language, construction and praxis, orientation, is widely used. However this remains an open research field.

As the ADAS-Cog is recorded on a categorical scale and response may be related to baseline in a non-linear manner, due consideration should be given to the appropriate analysis of treatment effects determined by changes from baseline.

2.2.2 Self care and activities of daily living

These measurements usually rely largely upon the reports of relatives or carers in close and regular contact with the patient.

ADL assessment is useful to evaluate the impact of a medicinal product-linked improvement in everyday functioning. Several scales have been proposed to measure either basic activities of daily living (or self-care) which relate to physical activities, such as toileting, mobility, dressing and bathing or instrumental activities of daily living, such as shopping, cooking, doing laundry, handling finances, using transportation, driving and phoning.

2.2.3 Global assessment

Global assessment refers to an overall subjective

independent rating of the patient's condition by a clinician experienced in the management of AD patients. Despite certain limitations, the clinician's global assessment can serve as a useful measure of the clinical relevance of a medicinal product's antidementia effect.

A global scale allows a single subjective integrative judgement by the clinician on the patient's symptoms and performance, as opposed to assessing various functions by means of a composite scale or a set of tests (see 2.2.4 Comprehensive assessment). Although a global assessment of patients benefit is less reliable than objective measurements of response and often appears insufficient to demonstrate by itself an improvement, it should be part of clinical trials in AD as it represents a way to validate results obtained in comprehensive scales or objective tests.

The Clinician's Interview Based Impression Of Change is recognised to be less responsive to drug effect than psychometric tests alone.

2.2.4 Comprehensive assessment

Comprehensive assessment is meant to measure and rate together in an additive way several domains of the illness, e.g. cognitive deficits, language deficits, changes in affect and impulse control. Scores proven to be useful in describing the overall clinical condition should be used, such as the Clinical Dementia Rating (CDR).

However, rather than composite scores derived from summing or averaging scores in different domains, the use of a set of instruments to quantify individually the dimensions of impairment, disability and handicap (social participation) should be encouraged.

2.2.5 Quality of life

Although quality of life is an important dimension of the consequences of diseases, the lack of validation of its assessment in AD does not allow specific recommendations to be made as yet. When adequate instruments to assess this dimension in patients and their caregivers become available, quality of life assessment may be justified in AD trials.

III GENERAL STRATEGY

The following recommendations apply mainly to AD but can be adapted to other forms of dementia (e.g. vascular dementia).

1 Phase I. Early pharmacology and pharmacokinetic studies

In the early phases of the development of antidementia medicinal products it is important to establish the pharmacological rationale on which the drug may be thought to be effective. Side effects and possible surrogate markers of pharmacological activity in volunteers, if available and relevant, might give some estimation of the appropriate dose.

Standard pharmocokinetic studies (see Note for

Guidance on Pharmacokinetic Studies in Man, Vol. III of The Rules Governing Medicinal Products on the European Union) must aim at defining the absorption, distribution, metabolism and elimination of the drug.

2 Phase II. Initial therapeutic trials

As it is difficult to seek improvement and probably unrealistic to expect recovery in advanced dementia, efficacy studies should be carried out mainly in patients suffering from mild or moderate forms of the disease. The inclusion of the same type of patients in Phases II and III should be advised, as safety issues may not be the same in different subgroups. Ideally such studies are carried out in the patient's everyday surroundings. These studies in well-characterised samples of demented patients have the following objectives:

- preliminary evaluation of efficacy
- assessment of short-term adverse reactions from a clinical and laboratory standpoint
- determination of pharmacokinetic characteristics
- definition of doses presumed to be effective
- determination of maximal tolerated doses.

The duration of such trials will depend either upon the time of response that is expected, or may be one of the parameters to be assessed.

3 Phase III. Controlled clinical trials

Symptomatic improvement studies have the following main objectives:

- demonstrating efficacy of the drug and estimating the temporal course and duration of such effects;
- assessing medium and long-term adverse effects.

Controlled clinical trials aimed at demonstrating short term improvement should last at least 6 months. Such studies should include placebo and/or comparators where appropriate. However studies of one year or more would be desirable to evaluate the maintenance of efficacy. The results of such extended studies might have an impact on labelling of compounds demonstrating efficacy.

Open label follow-up of at least 12 months are recommended for demonstrating long term safety. This can be achieved with an extension of the trial over the initially scheduled period in patients considered as responders and/or asking for continuing the treatment. In addition to responding adequately to an ethical issue, this allows to accumulate data on medium/long term safety of the drug and to estimate the maximal duration of the symptomatic effects.

Periodic evaluation of efficacy and safety should be performed at regular intervals, depending on the anticipated rapidity of action of the medicinal product and the duration of the trial. After the end of the treatment administration, the state of the patients should be followed for possible adverse events related to withdrawal treatment for a period appropriate for the drug being tested.

With regard to safety, as in the case of medicinal products designed for prolonged use (cf. Note for Guidance on Clinical Investigation of Medicinal Products for Long-Term use, Vol. III of The Rules Governing Medicinal Products in the European Union), at least 100 good quality cases of patients followed-up for 1 year or more should be available.

4 Adjustment for prognostic variables

Based on theoretical, experimental or observational considerations, the course of the disease and/or the efficacy of treatments may differ within subgroups of patients with AD or other dementias.

Some examples of prognostic factors to take into consideration could be as follows:

- Apo lipoprotein E genotype
- suspicion of Lewy body pathology (fluctuation of cognition, hallucinations, Parkinsonism);
- severity of dementia at inclusion;
- presence of vascular risk factors.

The factor(s) to be taken into account in the analysis should be identified in the protocol, the rationale should be given, and the study should be powered to yield a sufficient number of patients with or without the factor(s) to allow a statistically valid conclusion.

5 Concomitant treatments

In order to eliminate any interference or bias, it is desirable, particularly in Phase II trials to avoid any treatment likely to impair alertness, intellectual function and behaviour. These include hypnotic, anxiolytic, antidepressant, antipsychotic, anticholinergic and memory enhancing drugs. If they cannot be avoided, the acceptable level of use of such medicinal products should be set a priori in the protocol and remain constant throughout the trial.

Pharmacodynamic interaction studies between the test drug and the drugs commonly used in the elderly should be conducted, including psychotropic drugs used to control behavioural disturbances.

Address for correspondence

7 Westferry Circus
Canary Wharf
London E14 4HB
UK

mail@emea.eudra.org

www.eudra.org/emea.html

Canadian Guidelines for the Development of Anti-Dementia Therapies: A Conceptual Summary

Reference   Mohr E, Feldman H, Gauthier S (1995) Canadian guidelines for the development of antidementia therapies: a conceptual summary. *Canadian Journal of Neurological Sciences* 22: 62–71

Purpose

To provide guidelines on the development of anti-dementia therapy. The magnitude of the problem faced by Canadian society as a result of an ageing population has been identified. Perhaps the most important concern related to this greying of Canada is the incidence of dementia and Alzheimer's disease. Therapeutic options for these disorders have been limited to date. Advances in biotechnology and molecular biology will offer novel approaches to treatment. These, and the expansion of more traditional therapeutic avenues, require guidelines with the aim of optimizing their development.

Summary

The guidelines are essentially descriptive and follow the following domains: diagnosis; therapeutic design; phases of drug development; measurement; therapeutic approaches.

Address for correspondence
Dr Erich Mohr
Neuropsychology Lab
Room D733
Ottawa Civic Hospital
1053 Carling Avenue
Ottawa, Ontario
K1Y 4E9
Canada

Individualized Music Therapy

Reference   University of Iowa Gerontological Nursing Interventions Research Center, Research Dissemination Core 1996, updated 1999

Purpose

To describe strategies for alleviating agitation in confused elderly persons through the use of individualized music. The guideline is intended for use by nurses, and was developed based on a review of the literature in the area by a panel of experts.

Summary

Individualized music can be used for patients at risk or who are experiencing agitation or confusion. The music collection should be in accordance with the patient's preference, history and capacity to hear. Often an effect is achieved by implementing the intervention a minimum of 30 minutes prior to the patient's usual peak level of agitation. Ongoing assessment should be conducted to determine the patient's response to the music intervention. Other patients who are in close proximity to the music being played should be assessed in case the music may have an unintended negative effect on them. The patient should be monitored while the music is being played to ensure that the agitation does not increase the confusion, or the agitation does not become more pronounced.

Address for correspondence

University of Iowa Gerontological Nursing Interventions Research Center
Research Dissemination Core
4118 Westlawn
Iowa City, IA 52242-1009
USA

Practice Parameter: Management of Dementia (an Evidence-Based Review)

Reference   Doody RS, Steven JC, Beck C, Dubinsky RM, Kaye JA, Gwyther L, Mohs RC, Thal LJ, Whitehouse PJ, DeKosky ST, Cummings JL (2001) Practice parameter: management of dementia (an evidence-based review): report of the Quality Standards Subcommittee of the American Academy of Neurology. *Neurology* 56: 1154–66

Purpose

To define and investigate key issues in the management of dementia and to make literature based treatment recommendations. Four clinical questions were addressed.

1. Does pharmacotherapy for cognitive symptoms improve outcomes in patients with dementia?
2. Does pharmacotherapy for non-cognitive symptoms improve outcomes in patients with dementia?
3. Do educational interventions improve outcomes in patients and/or caregivers of patients with dementia compared with no such interventions?
4. Do nonpharmacologic interventions other than education improve outcomes in patients and/or caregivers of patients with dementia compared with no such interventions?

The classification of evident level of recommendations are the same as those for early detection of dementia.

Summary

1. Does pharmacotherapy for cognitive symptoms improve outcomes in patients with dementia compared with no therapy?

Conclusion

Significant treatment effects have been demonstrated with several different cholinesterase inhibitors indicating that the class of agents is consistently better than placebo. However, the disease eventually continues to progress despite treatment and the average effect size of treatment is modest. Global changes in cognition behaviour and functioning have been detected by both physicians and caregivers indicating that even small measurable differences may be clinically significant. To date, there have been no head to head comparisons of cholinesterase inhibitors and the main differences between these agents are in the side effect profiles and the ease of administration (e.g. once or twice versus four times daily dosing). Current studies do not support the efficacy of cholinergic precursors or muscarinic agonists for the treatment of Alzheimer's disease. It is unclear whether highly selective M1 agonists delivered in adequate doses to the CNS would be beneficial and tolerable in Alzheimer's disease. A wide group of agents with diverse mechanisms of action have been tested in at least one Class I trial. There is incomplete or conflicting

evidence for these agents. One study suggests a possible benefit of vitamin E or possibly Selegiline for the treatment of Alzheimer's disease. The agents should not be combined. The use of anti-inflammatory agents prednisone and estrogen to prevent the progression of Alzheimer's disease are not supported by prospective data. Gingko biloba was safe in one Class I trial of patients with mixed dementia but benefits fall short of those expected for clinically effective anti-dementia treatments (e.g. psychometric measure and a clinician's global score). Currently there are no adequately controlled trials supporting the use of any pharmacologic agents in patients believed to have mixed neurodegenerative and ischaemic vascular dementia or in populations in which the specific type of dementia is not identified.

Practice recommendations

Pharmacologic treatment of AD

- Cholinesterase inhibitors should be considered in patients with mild to moderate AD (Standard), although studies suggest a small average degree of benefit.
- Vitamin E (1000 I.U. PO BID) should be considered in an attempt to slow progression of AD (Guideline)
- Selegiline (5 mg PO BID) is supported by one study but has a less favourable risk-benefit ratio (Practice Option)
- There is insufficient evidence to support the use of other antioxidants, anti-inflammatories, or other putative disease-modifying agents specifically to treat AD because of the risk of significant side effects in the absence of demonstrated benefits (Practice Option)
- Estrogen should not be prescribed to treat AD (Standard)

Mixed populations or patients with mixed dementias,

- Some patients with unspecified dementia may benefit from ginkgo biloba, but evidence-based efficacy data are lacking (Practice Option)

Ischaemic vascular dementia

- There are no adequately controlled trials demonstrating pharmacologic efficacy for any agent in ischemic vascular (multi-infarct) dementia.

2. Does pharmacotherapy for noncognitive symptoms improve outcomes for patients with dementia and/or their caregivers compared with no therapy?

Class I evidence supports the use of both traditional and

atypical antipsychotics in the treatment of agitation and psychosis in dementia and atypical agents seem to be better tolerated. There is little evidence to support the use of other agents such as anticonvulsives, benzodiazapines, antihistamines, monoamine oxidase inhibitors or SSRIs for the treatment of agitation of psychosis in dementia or the treatment of depression. SSRIs may offer some benefit and better tolerability than other antidepressants.

Practice recommendations

- antipsychotics should be used to treat agitation or psychosis in patients with dementia where environmental manipulation fails (Standard). Atypical agents may be better tolerated compared with traditional agents (Guideline)
- Selected tricyclic, MAO-B inhibitors, and SSRI should be considered in the treatment of depression in individuals with dementia with side effect profiles guiding the choice of agent (Guideline).

3. Do educational interventions improve outcomes for patients with dementia and/or their caregivers compared with no interventions?

Conclusions

Evidence from Class I and III studies suggest that short-term educational programs are well liked by family caregivers and can lead to a modest increase in disease knowledge and greater confidence among caregivers. Extensive training for caregivers may lead to delayed nursing home placement. Educational training for staff of long-term care facilities can decrease the use of antipsychotic medications without increasing the rate of disruptive behaviors.

Practice recommendations

- short term programs directed toward educating family caregivers about Alzheimer's disease should be offered to improve caregiver satisfaction (Guideline)
- Intensive long-term education and support services (when available) should be offered to caregivers of patients with Alzheimer's disease to delay time to nursing home placement (Guideline)
- staff of long-term care facilities should receive education about Alzheimer's disease to reduce the use of unnecessary antipsychotics (Guideline).

4. Do nonpharmacologic interventions other than education improve outcomes for patients and their caregivers compared with no such interventions?

Two Class I studies show that behaviour modification, scheduled toileting and prompted voiding can reduce urinary incontinence. On Class I studies supported by Class II and Class III data shows that graded assistance skills practice and positive reinforcement can increase functional independence in persons with dementia. Sensory stimulation of various types (auditory, visual and tactile) are usually included as part of a complex multi-faceted approach so it is difficult to make conclusions about their efficacy. Psychosocial interventions directed towards patients may benefit them but the a priori outcome measures are often negative and the programs are not easily replicated. Therapeutic benefits of special environments were difficult to evaluate but may have a beneficial impact on agitation and psychosocial interventions directed towards caregivers including education, support and respite care may improve caregivers emotional well-being and quality of life and may delay nursing home placement for patients with dementia.

Practice recommendations
Functional performance

- Behavior modification schedules toileting and prompted voiding should be used to reduce urinary incontinence (Standard)
- Graded assistant, practice and positive reinforcement should be used to increase functional independence (Guideline)
- Low lighting levels, music and simulated nature sounds may improve eating behaviors for person with dementia, and intensive multimodality group training may improve activities of daily living, but these approaches lack conclusive supporting data (Practice Options)

Problem behaviors

- Persons with dementia may experience decreased problem behaviors with the following interventions: music, particularly during meals and bathing (Guideline); walking or other forms of light exercise (Guideline)
- Although evidence is suggestive only, some patients may benefit from the following (Practice Options):
  - simulated presence therapy, such as the use of videotaped or audiotaped family
  - massage
  - comprehensive psychosocial care programs
  - pet therapy
  - commands issued at the patient's comprehension level
  - bright light, white noise
  - cognitive remediation

Care environment alterations

- Although definitive data are lacking, the following environments may be considered for patients with dementia (Practice Options)
  - special care units (SCU) within long-term care facilities
  - homelike physical setting with small groups of patients as opposed to traditional nursing homes

- short-term, planned hospitalization of 1 to 3 weeks with or without blended inpatient and outpatient care

- provision of exterior space, remodeling corridors to simulate natural or home settings and changes in the bathing environment.

Interventions for caregivers

- the following interventions may benefit caregivers of persons with dementia and may delay long-term placement (Guidelines)

- comprehensive, psychoeducational caregiver training
- support groups

- additional patient and caregiver benefits may be obtained by use of computer networks to provide education and support to caregivers (Practice Option), telephone support programs (Practice Option), and adult day care for patients and other respite services (Practice Option).

Summary
175 references

Consensus Report of the Working Group on Molecular and Biochemical Markers of Alzheimer's Disease

Reference   (1998) Consensus Report of the Working Group on: 'Molecular and Biochemical Markers of Alzheimer's Disease'. *Neurobiology of Aging* 19: 109–16

Purpose

The Working Group had three goals: first, to define the characteristics of ideal biological markers; second, to outline the process whereby a biological marker gains acceptance in the medical and scientific communities; and third, to review the current status of all proposed biomarkers for Alzheimer's disease.

Summary

The recommended steps in the process of establishing a biomarker are:

1. There should be at least two independent studies that specify the biomarker's sensitivity, specificity, and positive and negative predictive values.
2. Sensitivity and specificity should be no less than 80 per cent, positive predictive value should approach 90 per cent.
3. The studies should be well powered, conducted by investigators with expertise to conduct such studies, and the results published in peer-reviewed journals.
4. The studies should specify the type of control subjects, including normal subjects and those with a dementing illness but not AD.
5. Once a marker is accepted, follow-up data should be collected and disseminated to monitor their accuracy and diagnostic value.

The review of current candidate markers indicates that for suspected early-onset familial AD, it is appropriate to search for mutations in the presenilin 1, presenilin 2 and amyloid precursor protein genes. Individuals with these mutations typically have increased levels of the amyloid $A\beta_{42}$ peptide in plasma and decreased levels of APPs in cerebrospinal fluid. In late-onset and sporadic AD these measures are not useful, but detecting an apolipoprotein E $\epsilon4$ allele can add confidence to the clinical diagnosis. Among the other proposed molecular and biochemical markers for sporadic AD, cerebrospinal fluid assays showing low levels of $A\beta_{42}$ and high levels of tau come closest to fulfilling criteria for a useful biomarker.

Address for correspondence

John H Growdon
Chair of the Working Group Advisory Committee
WACC 830
Massachusetts General Hospital
Boston, MA 02114
USA

Consensus Statement on Predictive Testing for Alzheimer's Disease

Reference   (1995) Consensus statement on predictive testing for Alzheimer's disease. *Alzheimers Disease and Associated Disorders* 94: 182–7

Purpose

To discuss predictive genetic testing for Alzheimer's disease.

Summary

Discussion revolved round a number of specific points: defining predictive testing; defining the outcome of predictive testing; the genetic contribution; apolipoprotein E; the differences between diagnostic testing and predictive testing; genetic screening of the population; experience from Huntington's disease (HD); the advantages and disadvantages of predictive testing for AD; and the ethical, scientific and clinical issues. The consensus was summarized in five main points:

1. Apart from a few rare families with early-onset FAD associated with the APP mutations, the time for presymptomatic predictive testing for AD in general has not yet arrived. Diagnostic testing may be clinically indicated, and genetic testing for research purposes, provided it falls within stringent ethical guidelines, remain important if the field is to progress.

2. When the time for clinical predictive testing arrives, guidelines previously developed for HD and adapted for AD (Lennox *et al*, 1994) may prove useful.

3. Further research into the molecular biology and genetics of AD is clearly important. This must include not only basic biological research, but also consideration of the psychosocial consequences of testing. International research, which is strongly supported by the ADI, may prove particularly revealing.

4. New findings should be published in refereed scientific journals. There is a need for informed debate about the issues raised. Dramatic public announcements of genetic breakthroughs that have not been exposed to informed scrutiny are best avoided, as they can be very disturbing to family members.

5. The five 'C's (consent, counselling, confidentiality, costs and consequences) remain the cornerstones of any testing procedure.

Consent requires the person undergoing testing to be aware of the implications and possible consequences of testing, and his or her rights, including the right not to have the test. Published recommendations for HD on predictive testing include the following: up-to-date relevant information should be available to the individual; the individual makes the decision about undertaking the test, and no third-party requests can be considered; and the individual must have reached the age of majority. Alzheimers associations have an important role in publicizing information about predictive testing.

Counselling requires access to a skilled, competent professional, usually within a specialized genetics unit, who is knowledgable about the tests and their meaning. It is recommended that a trusted partner, preferably one not at risk of AD, accompanies the individual. Current or past psychiatric illness may require postponement of testing or special counselling services.

Confidentiality must be as absolute as the country's laws allow, so that no one else apart from the affected person and the professionals involved is aware of the results of testing. No third party should ever be contacted or given any information regarding testing without written consent from the individual concerned.

Costs (both financial and psychological) of screening presymptomatic patients if there are no clinical indications must be weighed against the potential benefits in life planning and equanimity of mind. Individuals at significant risk or with a clinical indication should be able to undertake testing regardless of their financial means.

Consequences of testing require full discussion. These may be positive or negative, and may have effects on the extended family as well as on the person seeking the information.

Reference

Lennox A, Karlinsky H, Meschino W, Buchanan JA, Percy JA, Percy ME, Berg JM (1994) Molecular genetic predictive testing for Alzheimer's disease: deliberations and preliminary recommendations. *Alzheimers Disease and Associated Disorders* 8: 126–47.

Address for correspondence

Professor Henry Brodaty
Academic Department for Old Age Psychiatry
University of New South Wales
Prince of Wales Hospital
Randwick
NSW 2031
Australia

Statement on Use of Apolipoprotein E Testing for Alzheimer's Disease

Reference   American College of Medical Genetics/American Society of Human Genetics Working Group on ApoE and Alzheimer Disease (1995). Statement on use of Apolipoprotein E testing for Alzheimer Disease. *Journal of the American Medical Association* 274: 1627–9

Purpose

To evaluate the published data on the association between apolipoprotein E genotype and Alzheimer's disease, and determine whether the data support the use of genetic testing for prediction of disease.

Summary

The American College of Medical Genetics and the American Society of Human Genetics developed a ten-member working group to assess the available data, using peer-reviewed journal publications from an Index Medicus literature search. The main conclusions were that there is a general consensus that ApoE $\epsilon4$ is strongly associated with AD, and that when present it may represent an important risk factor for the disease. However, at the present time it is not recommended for use in routine clinical diagnosis, nor should it be used for predictive testing. Studies to date indicate that low genotyping to be used as a diagnostic test. Because AD develops in the absence of ApoE $\epsilon4$ and because many with ApoE $\epsilon4$ seem to escape disease, genotyping is also not recommended for use as a predictive genetic test. The results of a collaborative study underway will clarify some of these issues. Whether ApoE genotypes have other uses in the management of AD will become apparent over the next few years.

Address for correspondence

Lindsay Farrer
Dept of Neurology
Boston University School of Medicine
80E Concord Street
Boston, MA 02118-2394
USA

The Clinical Introduction for Genetic Testing for Alzheimer's Disease: An Ethical Perspective

Reference   Post SG, Whitehouse P, Binstock RH *et al* (1997) Consensus statement. The clinical introduction of genetic testing for Alzheimer disease: an ethical perspective. *Journal of the American Medical Association* 277: 832–6

Purpose

To provide physicians with guidelines to deal with the situation when they are approached to carry out genetic tests in relation to risk of Alzheimer's disease.

Summary

Several professional ethical questions are faced by physicians when approached about genetic testing in relation to Alzheimer's disease. First, for which patients and for what purpose is it clinically and ethically appropriate to introduce genetic testing for Alzheimer's disease? Second, how should demand for such testing be answered? Third, what standard should govern the disclosure of test results in the light of potential discrimination? To address these issues, a multidisciplinary national study group was created with the support of the National Institutes of Health to review emerging information on AD genetic testing. The group was composed of leading Alzheimer's geneticists, policy experts, and ethicisits, with input from patients with mild Alzheimer's disease and their caregivers.

The group considered both single gene disorder known to be implicated in the etiology of Alzheimer's disease as well as apolipoprotein E4, which is known to be a biological risk factor for the disorder. One of the main issues is that in the public mind apolipoprotein E4 has been confused with the autosomal dominant genes, with the assumption by many people that testing for E4 will achieve a result which is predictive of the development of Alzheimer's disease. The debate has taken a significant turn with these tests becoming widely available to the general public. With regard to genetic testing in the single gene dominant mutations, the analogy was drawn to the status for genetic testing for other autosomal dominant neurodegenerative diseases such as Huntington's disease. However, the point was made that it is highly likely that several autosomal dominant mutations that produce Alzheimer's disease have not been identified, and so a negative screen does not mean a mutation does not exist. With regard to apolipoprotein susceptability, five groups have developed consensus statements regarding genetic testing using apolipoprotein. The American College of Medical Genetics/American Society of Human Genetics Working Group concluded that ApoE genotypes' lack of sensitivity or specificity makes it inappropriate for use as a diagnostic or predictive test. The UK Alzheimer's Disease Genetics Consortium

concurred. The Medical and Scientific Advisory Committee of Alzheimer's Disease International expressed concern about the potential for misinforming patients about the risk. The National Institute on Ageing, The Alzheimer's Disease and Related Disorders Association issued a consensus statement leaving it to the physicians' discretion as to the diagnostic use of apolipoprotein E testing as an adjunct to established diagnostic tests. The Alzheimer's Disease and Related Disorders Association and National Ethics Advisory Panel issued a notice saying the apolipoprotein E genotyping should not be used in asymptomatic individuals. The view of the current consensus was that testing should be discouraged, although there are anecdotal reports to suggest it has been offered by some clinicians to especially demanding consumers who are willing to pay for it. When apolipoprotein E testing is done in the course of a medically indicated evaluation of serum lipid profiles for the management of cardiovascular disease, the patient should be prospectively informed of the supplemental information intrinsic to apolipoprotein E testing. The patient should be advised that this testing unavoidably determines whether a gene related to AD is present, that there may be implications for recording these data in the medical record, and that he or she has the option of having the AD implications of this testing discussed with him or her. A point which is also worth making is that, unlike the measurement of serum cholesterol or sugar, a test such as this may give genetic information to a son or daughter who may not wish it.

The conclusion is that, except for autosomal dominant early onset families, genetic testing in asymptomatic individuals is unwarranted. The use of apolipoprotein E as an adjunct to other diagnostic tests may be of benefit, but remains under investigation. The premature introduction of genetic testing and possible adverse consequences are to be avoided.

Address for correspondence

Dr Stephen Post
Center for Biomedical Ethics
School of Medicine
Case Western Reserve University
Cleveland, OH 44106
USA

Guidelines for Alzheimer's Disease Management

Reference California Workgroup on Guidelines for Alzheimer's Disease Management (1999). Guidelines for Alzheimer's Disease Management. Los Angeles Alzheimer's Association

Purpose

To serve as a general guide for the ongoing management of people with Alzheimer's disease, the intended audience being primary care practitioners including physicians, nurse practitioners, physician assistants, social workers and other professionals providing primary care. The work comes from the Standards Committee of the Alzheimer's Disease Diagnostic and Treatment Centres of California. Various headings are included.

Summary

Assessment

An assessment should be carried out of daily function (including feeding, bathing, dressing, mobility, toileting, continence and ability to manage finances and medications).

Cognitive status should be assessed using a reliable and valid instrument (e.g. the MMSE), other medical or behavioral problems, psychotic symptoms or depression with reassessment occurring every 6 months. Identify the primary care giver and assess the adequacy of family support and the decision making capacity of the patient.

Treatment recommendations are: to develop and implement an ongoing treatment plan of defined goals which include the use of cholinesterase inhibitors; referral to appropriate structured activities such as exercise, recreation and adult day care; appropriate treatment of medical conditions; to treat behavioral problems and mood disorders with non-pharmacological approaches and referral to social service agencies or support organizations; medications if clinically indicated.

Recommendations

It is recommended that the diagnosis and progression of Alzheimer's disease is discussed with the patient and family in a manner consistent with their values and preferences and the patient's abilities. It is also recommended that there is referral to support organizations for education materials, community resources, support groups, legal and financial issues, respite care, future care needs and options. Furthermore, is it suggested that there is discussion regarding the patient's need to make advance directives and to identify surrogates for medical and legal decision-making.

Reporting requirement

1. Abuse – (monitor for evidence and report all instances to adult protective services or police department as required by law).
2. Driving – report diagnosis of AD in accordance with California law.

Address for correspondence

Los Angeles Alzheimer's Association
5900 Wilshire Blvd
Suite 1710
Los Angeles, CA 90036
USA

www.alzla.org

Guidelines for the Support and Management of People with Dementia

Reference   National Advisory Committee on Health and Disability Services: Wellington, New Zealand (1997)

Purpose

The guidelines are targeted at primary health care practitioners and represent the first stage in developing best practice advice for people with dementia (the next stage was to work with the Alzheimer Society and general practitioners to develop a practical, accessible summary document for general practitioners).

Summary

- People with dementia and their carers need continuity of well co-ordinated care throughout the span of the illness.
- As general practitioners are often the first point of contact for services, it is vital that there is consistency of diagnostic criteria and prompt access to specialist advice available for those cases which require it.
- General practitioners should be conversant with appropriate referral and information services.
- Every New Zealand citizen should have access, when necessary, to expert specialist advice on dementia from a publicly funded service.
- There should be nationwide uniformity of Elder Abuse Services, and each region of the country should have a publicly funded elder abuse team.
- Carers must have specific information and counselling for emotional problems throughout the illness.
- Carers need services that are timely, appropriate and individually planned.
- Implementation of standardized, mandatory training in dementia for all medical students in both the pre-clinical and clinical years.
- Implementation of standardized, mandatory training in dementia for all nursing staff, ancillary staff, and allied health professionals at undergraduate level.
- National implementation of these guidelines for dementia, including specific training in service contracts with residential care facilities, in particular those providing specialized dementia care.
- Training programmes for family carers should be available throughout the country, resourced by RHAs.
- Appropriate funding for the Alzheimer's Society's administration of its national awareness and information programmes should be made available.
- Government policy and funding should recognize the importance of trained careworkers, and require and resource the RHAs to ensure funding for training and adequate payment of trained staff is built into service contracts.
- Dementia-specific services should be appropriately recognized and publicly funded.
- New Zealand data on the economic costs of dementia care and research into care innovations are urgently required.
- Information about the Protection of Personal Property and Rights Act 1988 should be freely available to health care professionals and carers. Consideration should be given to distribution of a refresher package.

The contents include:

1. Introduction
2. Definition
3. Incidence and prevalence of dementia in New Zealand
4. The clinical spectrum of dementia, diagnosis
5. Diagnosis
6. Cognition enhancing drug treatments
7. Management of dementia
8. Community care
9. Cultural issues
10. Recommendations for research
11. Audit of care for persons with dementia

and a number of appendices with details of specific instruments, a note of costs of dementia care and the role of investigations.

Address for correspondence

Professor Richard Sainsbury
Health Care of the Elderly
Christchurch School of Medicine
PO Box 4345
Christchurch
New Zealand

www.nzgg.org.nz/library/gl_complete/dementia/index.cfm
contents

Dementia in the Community: Management Strategies for General Practice

Reference   Alzheimer's Disease Society UK (1999)

Purpose

To help GPs and primary care team colleagues to identify, diagnose and manage dementia in the community.

Summary

The guide is divided into a number of chapters: What is dementia?; The role of the GP; Diagnosis: The needs of the person with dementia; The needs of the carer; Management of common problems; Framework for good practice; Issues for further discussion; Appendices.

The guide is designed to help general practitioners and their primary health care team colleagues to:

- stimulate earlier identification of cases to help the patient and carer to come to terms with the diagnosis and prognosis
- provide an easy method of assessment to enable the primary health care team to make collaborative plans for future services
- reach the correct diagnosis and detect any remedial pathology
- carry out a review of the patients' medication

- assess the patient's functional state and encourage optimum functioning
- anticipate and avert crises by assessing social and domestic circumstances
- trigger the provision of social support and make appropriate referrals to other agencies
- examine the needs of carers and find ways of providing them with information and advice for the future.

Addresses for correspondence

Alzheimer's Society
Gordon House
10 Greencoat Place
London, SW1P 1PH
UK

Alzheimer Scotland – Action on Dementia
8 Hill Street
Edinburgh, EH2 3JZ
UK

Guidelines for Care of Alzheimer's Disease

Reference   Fisk JD, Sadovnick D, Cohen CA, Gauthier S, Dossetor J, Eberhart A, Le Duc L (1998). *Canadian Journal of Neurological Sciences* 25: 242–8.

Purpose

The guidelines for care were developed in response to the need for national direction to ensure that people with Alzheimer's disease receive the special type of care that serves the unique nature of this disease. These guidelines are based on the assumption that all older adults, regardless of circumstances, are entitled to quality care.

Summary

The guidelines highlight the following areas:

1. *Training and education for caregivers:* this should be available to help them understand the disease process and assist them in their role as caregivers. Staff facilities and agencies should be required to participate in training and educational programs on meeting the needs of people with Alzheimer's disease and their carers.

2. *Support for caregivers:* the guidelines recognize that all services should meet the needs of family caregivers because of the significant burden and stress produced by the illness. All caregivers should have access to support and resources for relief of stress that may result from caring for a person with Alzheimer's disease.

3. *Individualized assessment:* each individual should receive comprehensive assessment that identifies his/her strengths, needs and abilities, and personal characteristics. Where possible the assessment should be carried out by a multidisciplinary team and should also address the social circumstances of the person with Alzheimer's disease and his or her caregivers. The assessment process should address the safety and security of the person with Alzheimer's disease, and ongoing assessment should monitor changes in the individual and in his/her circumstances.

4. *Individualized care planning for the individual with Alzheimer's disease:* this should be carried out by a multidisciplinary team and an individualized and comprehensive care plan should be prepared for each individual.

5. *Programs and activities:* programs for persons with Alzheimer's should include the routines of daily living as well as special activities. Programs serving people with Alzheimer's should promote wellbeing and enjoyment and programs with activities should be flexible and change in response to the changing needs of the person with Alzheimer's disease.

6. *Specialized human resources:* procedures relating to staff and volunteers working with dementia patients should reflect the special requirements of people with Alzheimer's disease. Performance appraisal should address the special issues facing staff and volunteers who provide care for people with Alzheimer's disease.

7. *Support and physical design:* the environment should meet the safety and security requirements of the individual with Alzheimer's disease. The environment should reduce the confusion of the person with Alzheimer's disease, and it should contribute to the effective functioning of the individual with Alzheimer's disease and their caregivers.

8. *Transportation:* this should be provided in a manner which ensures the safety and emotional comfort of the person with Alzheimer's disease.

9. *Decision making:* respecting individual choice: the individual with Alzheimer's disease and/or a designated decision maker should have maximum involvement when decisions about the person with Alzheimer's disease are taking place. If an assessment of competency is required, the assessment should be undertaken by an individual or team which has special training in making competency assessments.

10. *Prevention and response to abuse:* the emphasis should be on preventing abuse by identifying and alleviating circumstances which are likely to lead to physical, psychological or financial abuse or neglect. Facilities and agencies should have protocols that deal with abuse and caregivers should take action when they suspect abuse has occurred.

11. *Use of restraints:* the emphasis should be on eliminating the need to contemplate restraint use by preventing and managing the behavior which leads to the desire to use restraints. Each facility or agency should have a clearly stated protocol on the use of physical, chemical and environment restraints. Every effort should be made to reduce the negative impact of the experience and to preserve the person's dignity.

Address for correspondence

John Fisk PhD
Alzheimer's Society of Canada
20 Eglinton Avenue W
Suite 1200
Toronto, Ontario
M4R 1K8
Canada
http://www.alzheimer.ca

North of England Evidence-based Guideline Development Project for the Primary Care Management of Dementia

Reference   Eccles M, Clarke J, Livingstone M, Freemantle N, Mason J (1998) North of England evidence-based guidelines development project: guideline for the primary care management of dementia *British Medical Journal* 317: 802–8

Purpose

To provide recommendations to assist general practitioners to manage people with all forms of dementia and to help their carers. The guideline is available in summary.

Summary

The strength of recommendations were based on category of evidence:

I.   Well-designed randomized controlled trial, meta-analyses or systematic reviews
II. Well-designed cohort or case-controlled study
III. Uncontrolled studies or external consensus

Strength of recommendation where:

(a) based directly on category 1 evidence;
(b) directly based on category 2 evidence or extrapolated recommendation from category 1 evidence;
(c) directly based on category 3 evidence or extrapolated recommendation from category 1 or 2 evidence; and
(d) based on the group's clinical opinion.

Recommendations and important points were given in a number of different categories: prevalence, identifying people with dementia, physical screening in dementia, dementia of Lewy body type, depression in patients with dementia, non-psychotic behavioural disorders, falls, leaving home, non-drug therapy – residential care, drug treatment, carers.

Summary of recommendations

Aim and scope of the guideline

The aim of this guideline is to provide recommendations, to aid primary health care professionals in their management of people with dementia and their carers.

All recommendations are for primary health care professionals and apply to patients attending general practice with dementia. The development group assumes that health care professionals will use general medical knowledge and clinical judgement in applying the general principles and specific recommendations of this document to the management of individual patients.

Recommendations may not be appropriate for use in all circumstances. Decisions to adopt any particular recommendation must be made by the practitioner in the light of available resources and circumstances presented by individual patients.

Prevalence

Health care professionals should be aware of the increased incidence and prevalence of dementia with increasing age (B)

Health care professionals should be aware that complaints of subjective memory impairment are not a good indicator of dementia. A history of loss of function is more indicative (than memory impairment) (B)

Population screening for dementia in the over 65s is not recommended. A case finding approach is recommended (B)

Identifying people with dementia

The patient or carer's history

Health care professionals should be aware of the diminution of insight as dementia progresses, making the patient's history less reliable (B)

Because of the potential unreliability of the patient's history, in the assessment of a person with cognitive impairment a history of memory problems should be sought from a carer as well as the patient (B)

Health care professionals should be sensitive to the possible coexistence of dementia and other psychiatric symptomatology (delusions and/or hallucinations, usually persecutory in nature and simple in type) (B)

The General Practitioner

General Practitioners should consider the use of formal cognitive testing to enhance their clinical judgement (B)

Short Screening Tests for cognitive impairment

Health care professionals should consider the use of the following instruments as tools in helping to identify cognitive impairment (B):

- The Mini Mental State Examination
- The clock drawing test
- An instrument for assessing activities of daily living, e.g. CAPE
- Abbreviated Mental Test Score (C)

Physical screening of people with dementia in Primary Care

Health care professionals should be aware of the existence of reversible causes of dementia (B)

Health care professionals should be aware that people

with dementia experience physical morbidity to the same degree as the general population but are likely to under-report their symptoms (B)

General Practitioners should ensure that the following routine tests are performed: haematology (including Erythrocyte Sedimentation Rate), biochemistry, bone chemistry, thyroid function and simple urinalysis (B)

Dementia with Lewy Bodies

Health care professionals should be aware of the importance of differentially diagnosing Dementia with Lewy Bodies because of the high risk of increased morbidity and mortality with neuroleptic agents in these patients (B)

Depression in patients with dementia

Health care professionals should have a high index of suspicion for diagnosing depression in patients with dementia at any stage in the dementing process (C)

The history from patients assessed for depression should be gathered from both the patients and their carers (C)

Consider relevant risk factors for depressive illness such as personal or family history of depression or recent adverse events such as bereavement or relocation (C)

Consider a trial of anti-depressant medication at a therapeutic dose evaluated against explicit criteria such as activities of daily living, level of functioning, behavioural disturbance, biological features of recent onset (B)

Behavioural disorders in patients with dementia

Health care professionals should exclude underlying causes of behavioural disorder e.g. an acute physical illness, environmental distress or physical discomfort (D)

Where underlying causes are identified they should be managed before prescribing for the behavioural disorder (D)

General practitioners should, wherever possible, resist the routine use of tranquillisers to control behaviour disorders in patients in dementia (D)

In crisis situations the short term use of neuroleptics may be appropriate (D)

Patients known to have Dementia with Lewy Bodies should not be treated with neuroleptics (B)

There is a relationship between delusions and aggressive behaviour. Aggressive behaviour should be assessed with this in mind (D)

Health care professionals should be aware that the care setting and the attitudes of carers (or care teams in an institutional setting) may influence the emergence of behavioural problems (D)

Falls

Health care professionals should be aware that falls are increased in people with dementia (B)

Health care professionals should be aware of the factors contributing to the risk of falls which are medication, wandering and reversible confusion (B)

Health care professionals should be aware that people with dementia who fall are more likely to fall again (B)

Health care professionals should be aware that the risk of falls is not associated with the severity of the dementia but with the functional capability of the person, the risk being increased in the more capable group (B)

Leaving your own home

Health and social care professionals should be aware that the following factors are known to increase the likelihood of people with dementia having to leave their own homes: carer stress, physical dependence, irritability, nocturnal wandering and incontinence (B)

Health and social care professionals should be aware that the patient should not be assessed for optimal home care independently of the carer (B)

Non-drug therapies in dementia – residential care

Primary Health Care professionals should consider the use of structured programmes to encourage continuing independence for people with dementia resident in Nursing Homes (A)

Anti-dementia therapy

Aspirin in vascular dementia

Health care professionals should be aware that a reduction in risk of further vascular events for people who have early dementia known to be related to cerebral ischaemia may be achieved by treating with aspirin (75 mg); the size of any effect on cognitive impairment is unclear (B)

Health care professionals should be aware that stroke is a significant risk factor in the development of vascular dementia (A)

Hydergine

Hydergine is not sufficiently effective to be routinely recommended as a treatment for dementia (A)

Vasodilators

Vasodilators should not be prescribed as a treatment for dementia (A)

Tacrine

In the light of current knowledge tacrine should not be used by general practitioners for the treatment of dementia (A)

Donepezil Hydrochloride

In the light of limited current knowledge, general practitioners should not initiate treatment with donepezil (Aricept) (A)

In the light of limited current knowledge, general practitioners should not continue hospital initiated treatment with donepezil (Aricept) (A)

Carers

Care of the carers

Health care professionals should be aware that referral of carers to groups for the provision of support and information about dementia is valued by the carer although unlikely to reduce the carer burden (A)

Health care professionals should be aware that referral of patients to respite services offers satisfaction and relief of carers, though does not appear to alter the overall well being of the carer (A)

Health care professionals should be aware that referral of care recipients to respite and day care services may allow them to stay in their own home for longer (B)

Health care professionals should be aware that depressive illness is common in carers of people with dementia and is influenced by behavioural problems and higher care needs in the care recipient (B)

Health care professionals can improve satisfaction for carers by acknowledging and dealing with their distress and providing more information on dementia (C)

Impact of caring on caregivers

Health care professionals should be aware of the impact of caring for a person with dementia and the effect this has on the caregiver (B)

Health care professionals should be aware of the many factors contributing to the impact of caring and that male carers are less likely to complain spontaneously (B)

Health care professionals should be aware that the impact of caring is dependent not on the severity of the cognitive impairment but on the presentation of the dementia, e.g. factors such as behaviour and affect (B)

Available from: Department of Primary Care and Centre for Health Services Research, University of Newcastle upon Tyne, Newcastle upon Tyne NE2 4AA, UK.

Address for correspondence

Professor Martin Eccles
Dept of Primary Care and Centre for Health Services Research
University of Newcastle upon Tyne
Newcastle upon Tyne NE2 4AA
UK

Martin.Eccles@ncl.ac.uk

The Recognition, Assessment and Management of Dementing Disorders

Reference   Patterson CJ, Gauthier S, Bergman H, Cohen CA, Feightner JW, Feldman H, Hogan DB (1999) The recognition, assessment and management of dementing disorders: conclusions from the Canadian Consensus Conference on Dementia. *Canadian Medical Association Journal* 160 (Suppl 12): 1–15

Purpose

To build clinical practice guidelines for a primary care physician towards the recognition, assessment and management of dementing disorders. Forty-eight recommendations were put forward, addressing a variety of aspects of dementia care.

Summary

1. A detailed history and physical examination, including psychometric tests. In addition, scales looking at functional ability are needed and serial assessments over time may be necessary to establish a diagnosis.
2. For people with typical presentation, the only laboratory tests should be complete blood count, thyroid function tests, electrolytes, calcium and glucose.
3. A cranial CT is recommended if one or more of the following criteria are present: age under 60; rapid decline in cognitive function; short duration of dementia (less than 2 years); recent and significant head injury; unexplained neurological symptoms; history of cancer; use of anticoagulants; incontinence and gait disorder; new localizing signs; unusual or atypical cognitive symptoms; gait disturbance.
4. There is insufficient evidence to suggest that family physicians should use ancillary tests.
5. Most patients can be managed by their primary care physician. Referral to a geriatrician, geriatric psychiatrist, neurologist or other professional might be considered when there is:
   (a) continuing uncertainty about the diagnosis
   (b) a request by patient or family
   (c) the presence of depression
   (d) treatment problems, failure of medication
   (e) the need for additional help or caregiver support
   (f) the need to involve other health professionals
   (g) genetic counselling
   (h) for research studies.
6. Screening for cognitive impairment in the absence of symptoms of dementia is not recommended.
7. Screening in case finding is not recommended.
8. Family physician must have a high index of suspicion for dementia.
9. Memory complaints should be evaluated and the patient followed up.
10. Caregivers' reports of cognitive decline should be taken seriously.
11. Screening asymptomatic people for genetic risk factors is not recommended.
12. Genotyping in primary care is not recommended.
13. Attention should be paid to changes in people with Down's syndrome, as they are at high risk.
14. Referral to genetic counselling indicated if the family history is suggestive of autosomal dominance.
15. If a person with Alzheimer's disease is concerned about other family members, those relatives should be encouraged to consult their own doctors.
16. Consider collecting a blood sample for provincial DNA banking.
17. Control of number of conditions may prevent dementia.
18. Physicians should be aware of risk factors for Alzheimer's disease, such as genetic, substandard education, or head trauma.
19. NSAIDs cannot be recommended for the treatment or prevention of Alzheimer's disease.
20. The use of estrogen solely to prevent dementia is not recommended.
21. The diagnosis of dementia should be disclosed to the patient and family.
22. The physician should consider risks associated with driving.
23. Driving difficulties may indicate other problems.
24. Cessation of driving should be encouraged where appropriate.
25. Primary care physicians should notify licensing bodies of concern regarding competence to drive.
26. Validated performance-based driving assessments should be available.
27. Acknowledge the important role played by caregivers in dementia.
28. Educate the patients and families about the disease.
29. Evaluate caregiver coping strategies.
30. Assess caregivers' social support system.
31. Enquire about caregiver burden.
32. Refer caregivers to appropriate community services.
33. Discuss legal and financial issues with caregivers.
34. Family physicians should be aware of the cultural importance of families' recognition and acceptance of dementia.
35. Physicians should recognize that measures of cognitive function will often overestimate cognitive impairment in many cultural and linguistic groups.
36. Carer management of patients' specific cultures should be taken into account.
37. Physicians should consider diagnosing depression if the history is weeks rather than months or years.
38. Depressive illness should be treated and the patient may be referred to a specialist.

39. Treatment of mild depression should be non-pharmacological to begin with.
40. Emotional lability should be treated with an antidepressant mood stabilizer.
41. Enquiries should be made about behavioral and psychological symptoms of dementia.
42. Low doses of neuroleptics, an SSRI or trazodone should be prescribed for agitation.
43. Trazodone should be suggested for sleep disturbance.
44. Drugs should be regularly re-evaluated for their continuing need, and withdrawal considered.
45. Guidelines for antidementia drugs should be followed.
46. A trial course of donepezil should be prescribed for appropriate patients.
47. The use of vitamin E should not be recommended for the treatment and/or prevention of Alzheimer's disease (a dissenting minority opinion in favor of Vitamin E was added as an appendix to the report).
48. There is insufficient evidence to recommend ginkgo biloba.

Address for correspondence

Dr Christopher Patterson
Division of Geriatric Medicine
Hamilton Health Services Corporation
Chedoke Hospital Campus
Sanatorium Road
Hamilton, Ontario
L8N 3Z5
Canada

Privacy of Clients: Electronic Tagging and Closed-Circuit TV

Reference   UK Royal College of Nursing (1994)

Purpose

The use of closed-circuit television (CCTV) or electronic tagging is now widely debated in the health service, as to whether it is an unwarranted invasion of people's privacy or an acceptable way of reducing risk of accident. The RCN produced this position statement after an emergency resolution at its annual congress and in response to many inquiries from nurses.

Summary

The statement describes methods of CCTV and tagging together with the arguments for and against their use.
   Suggested guidelines:

1. A policy on electronic surveillance, agreed with staff and relatives, should be produced prior to it being implemented in a ward or unit.
2. Electronic surveillance should only be used as a short-term measure initially, and evaluated regularly thereafter.
3. If the purpose of surveillance and restraint is to prevent accidents, it could be that a compromise can be found. An 'acceptable level of risk' can then be negotiated between patients, relatives and health care staff.
4. Electronic surveillance should be documented in the nursing notes, and subject to continuous assessment and regular evaluation.
5. Electronic surveillance is no substitute for good nursing care. It should never be used to disguise inadequate staffing levels.
6. More appropriate alternatives to CCTV or tagging should be investigated first. A movement sensor would alert nurses to patients being up and about, or an audio alarm could transmit the noise of a fall or cry for help.

Address for correspondence

Royal College of Nursing
20 Cavendish Square
London SW1M 0AB
UK

Restraint Revisited – Rights, Risk and Responsibility: Guidance for Nurses Working with Older People

Reference   UK Royal College of Nursing (1999)

Purpose

The use of restraint is always an emotive issue. This revised guidance aims to stimulate a reasoned debate about the use and abuse of restraint, focusing on rights, risk and responsibility, rather than control and restraint. It supersedes earlier guidance, *Focus on Restraint*, published in 1992.

Summary

1. Restraint is defined as restricting liberty, preventing people from doing something they want to do. It is an intervention that prevents them from behaving in ways that threaten or cause harm to themselves, others or to property.

2. Every citizen not subject to legal detention has the right to be free from the use of unauthorized force, so anyone being restrained is being denied a fundamental human right, though there may at times be other overriding considerations. Anyone who applies any form of restraint should be prepared to justify the reason for doing so, but if this was the only way to prevent harm to the individual or others, and was for a short time, it is unlikely to be unlawful. Under certain circumstances, e.g. detention under the Mental Health Act, nurses may be empowered by law to use restraint.

3. Various methods of restraint may be employed, including locks, bedrails, harnesses, chairs, medication, isolation, electronic surveillance and staff behaviour. Restraint, if overused, can lead to a cycle of dependence. There may also be practical dangers; for example, pressure sores, incontinence and increased side effects of medication.

4. Nurses have a duty of care guided by the principles of beneficence, non-maleficence, justice and autonomy. Their practice is influenced by local guidelines and procedures, involvement of relatives in decisions, and informed consent, but they must put the wellbeing of the client first. This requires personal care plans and formal multidisciplinary reviews of care. Looking at the reasons behind clients' behaviour is an important first step, and often simple solutions can be found which lessen challenging behaviour and reduce the need for restraint.

5. Similar principles and considerations apply to working with clients in the community, either with informal carers or in residential and nursing homes.

6. In deciding to use restraint, nurses and their colleagues must assess and record why restraint is necessary, and monitor its use closely. Restraint must be a last resort and should only be considered when alternative methods of therapeutic behaviour management have failed.

Additional reference

Royal College of Nursing & NHS Executive (1998) *Safer Working in the Community: A Guide for NHS Managers and Staff on Reducing the Risks from Violence and Aggression.* RCN.

Address for correspondence

Royal College of Nursing
20 Cavendish Square
London SW1M 0AB
UK

European Transnational Alzheimer's Study (ETAS)

Reference   Warner M, Furnish S, Lawlor B, Longley M, Sime C, Kellet M (1998) European Transnational Alzheimer's Study (ETAS). European Analysis of Public Health Policy Developments for Alzheimer's Disease and Associated Disorders of Older People and Their Carers: Welsh Institute for Health and Social Care. ISBN: 1 84054 0033

Purpose

This was a study funded by the European Commission (DG5). Its aims were to explore the working definition of cognitive impairment across Europe, and to investigate the relationship of the definition of cognitive impairment in elderly people to policy and practice across Europe.

Summary

The following key issues and recommendations formed the basis of the report:

1. Alzheimer's sufferers and their carers are treated inequitably by member states.
2. There is inequity between and within member states in dealing with Alzheimer's disease.
3. Intervention often occurs at too late a stage in the progress of Alzheimer's disease.
4. Alzheimer's disease policy should be co-ordinated and services multidisciplinary.
5. Carers of Alzheimer's sufferers require better support.

Recommendations

1. There should be a concerted attempt both at national and European levels to use the most effective means of public education to change negative attitudes towards Alzheimer's disease and in particular to emphasize the benefits to be derived from early diagnosis.
2. Member states should use whatever policy levers they have available to increase the professional status of health care staff working with demented patients, and professional bodies themselves should develop strategies to achieve the same ends.
3. As part of the strategy to raise the status of AD services, member states should encourage the development of local, regional and national communities of interest for Alzheimer's disease that bring together all the relevant stakeholders. The commission should consider providing a degree of European co-ordination to such efforts.
4. The commission should work with member states to provide assistance to those whose services for Alzheimer's disease are at a less than ideal level of provision.
5. Member states should review and where necessary improve the consistency of local application of nationally accepted and community-wide good practice in relation to Alzheimer's disease.
6. The relevant bodies in each member state should develop an effective strategy to increase the level and quality of assessment and diagnosis of Alzheimer's disease at the early stages of the disease, and should consider setting targets to this end.
7. Each member state should also ensure that general medical and allied professional education includes sufficient input on dementia at undergraduate, postgraduate and continuing education levels.
8. Member states should continue to address the need to improve co-ordination at the policy and implementation levels to meet the total needs of Alzheimer's disease patients and their carers.
9. The boundaries between generalist and specialist provisions should be revised in each member state in order to ensure that both are fulfilling their most appropriate roles.
10. A mechanism should be established to evaluate and disseminate across Europe new models of service delivery and education.
11. There should be further improvements in the systematic identification of the needs of carers, supported by the allocation of adequate resources to meet their often modest requirements.
12. All member states should continue to improve the mechanisms used to involve caregivers in the planning of services.

Addresses for correspondence

Professor B Lawlor
Mercer's Institute on Ageing
St James's Hospital
Dublin 8
Ireland
e-mail: psychel@indigo.ie

Professor M Warner
The Welsh Institute for Health and Social Care
University of Glamorgan
Pontypridd CF37 1DL
UK

Guidelines for the Management of Agitation in Dementia

Reference   Ballard C, O'Brien J, Howard R (in press). UK Group for Optimization of Management of Alzheimer's Disease and other Dementias. Guidelines for the management of agitation in dementia. *International Journal of Geriatric Psychiatry*

Purpose

Agitation is a term describing excessive motor activity with a feeling of inner tension, characterized by such manifestations as anxiety and irritability, motor restlessness and abnormal vocalization. Behaviours such as pacing, wandering, aggression, shouting and night-time disturbance may occur. Agitation in dementia may have several causes, either related to the dementia (pain, other physical problems) or arising from the dementia (e.g. reactions to the patient's subjective experience). Agitated patients with dementia are often inappropriately given sedative drugs as first-line treatment, which may worsen the situation or produce serious side effects. This guidance is produced on behalf of a multidisciplinary group of specialists involved in the care of people with dementia in the UK.

Summary

Full and careful assessment of possible physical, psychological and environmental factors is essential. If no reversible physical cause is identified, minor degrees of agitation are often self-limiting and likely to resolve.

For agitation requiring further treatment, the following structured sequential approach is recommended:

1. The quality of care available to the patient should be optimized to ensure that facilities and available skills meet the patient's needs.
2. Non-pharmacological management should be tried first, and should be the mainstay of the treatment of agitation. This may comprise either a specifically tailored intervention aimed at the precipitants and reinforcers of the agitation, or more general brief structured intervention techniques, such as social interaction, activity, exercise, music or video/audio tapes of family members.
3. Pharmacological management may be indicated when other strategies have failed. The following points should be remembered:
   - there is no evidence from controlled trials to support the use of benzodiazepines
   - the use of antispychotics must involve consideration of risks as well as benefits
   - older people are sensitive to the common side effects of antipsychotics
   - there may be accelerated cognitive decline and sensitivity in dementia with Lewy bodies
   - there is modest evidence of efficacy for antipsychotic drugs
   - there are no demonstrated differences in efficacy, but atypical agents seem better tolerated
   - begin with lowest prescribable dose and carefully monitor for side effects
   - only continue medication if there is evidence of efficacy
   - review the continued need for treatment every 3 months
   - for patients where antipsychotics are ineffective or not tolerated, carbamazepine and trazodone may be efficacious
   - severe or treatment-resistant agitation merits specialist referral.

Address for correspondence

Dr Rob Howard
Section of Old Age Psychiatry
Institute of Psychiatry
De Crespigny Park
Denmark Hill
London SE5 8AF
UK

Treatment of Agitation in Older Persons with Dementia: A Special Report

Reference   Alexopoulos GS, Silver JM, Kahn DA *et al* (1998) *Postgraduate Medicine*

Purpose

The guidelines offer practical reference not only for clinicians but also for administrators, mental health educators and other health care professionals involved in the care of patients who have dementia. They offer a one-stop reference guideline of employing survey techniques and reflect the most current clinical standards. The guidelines take raters through the initial diagnosis of agitation and offer guidance for the overall and long-term management, from environmental intervention to suggested medication. The specific syndromes of agitation, including delirium, psychosis, depression, anxiety, insomnia, sundowning, aggression, anger and pain, are outlined in detail. Initial and secondary options are presented for each syndrome, along with advice regarding multiple nurses, single drug therapy, side effects and inadequate response to therapy. There is a section for families and caregivers. The survey questioned 100 leading experts in agitation and dementia, giving them 33 clinical situations and asking them to score on a scale from 1–9 the appropriateness of a particular intervention. Specific guidelines are offered with details on specific drug therapy, an algorithm for management strategies for agitation, preferred medications for subtypes of delirium, and the differential diagnosis of delirium.

Summary

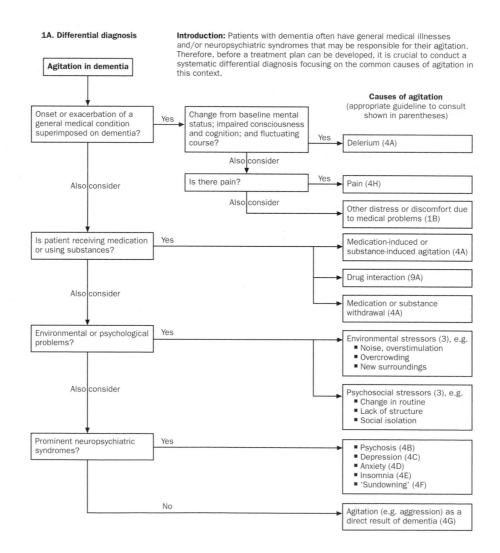

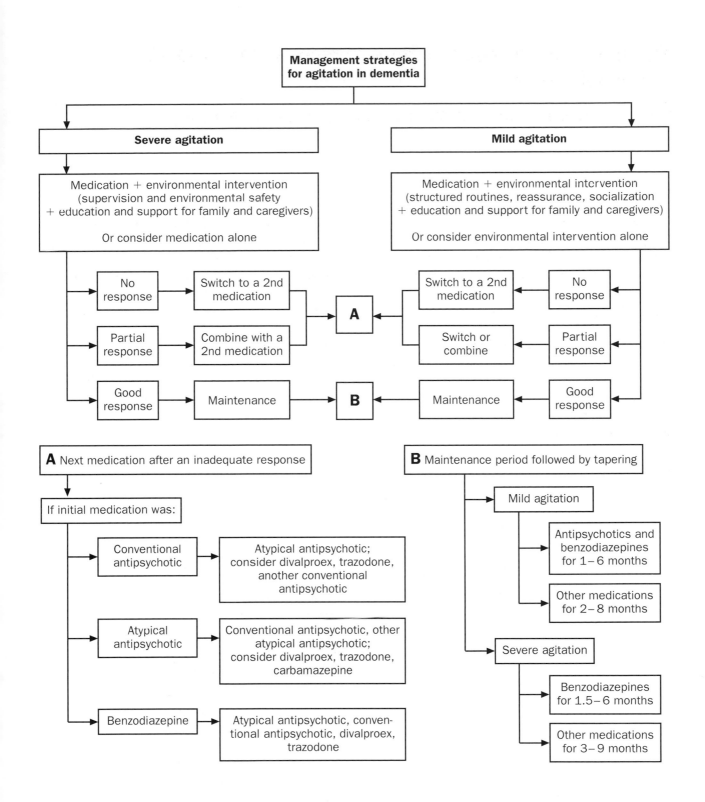

Address for correspondence

Healthcare Information Programs
McGraw-Hill Healthcare Information Group
4530 West 77th Street
Minneapolis, MN 55435
USA

Interventions in the Management of Behavioural and Psychological Aspects of Dementia

Reference   Scottish Inter-Collegiate Guidelines Network (SIGN) (1998) Edinburgh

Purpose

To make recommendations for the management of behavioural and psychological symptoms of dementia (BPSD). The guidelines review drug and non-drug interventions, giving each a grade of recommendation, a, b, or c (see summary and Quick Reference Guide). The rationale is that it is to allow the production of guidelines (primarily for use in Scotland), and is not meant to be taken as a standard of medical care.

Summary

The information on which the suggestions were made was based on a shortlist of about 3000 papers identified using a Medline and Embase search over 15 years up to September 1996, as well as information from Psychological Abstracts and the Cochrane database. The guidelines are split into different chapters, including the general assessment of dementia, issues of consent, recommendations for further research, and specific chapters on non-drug interventions, neuroleptic drugs and other drugs.

See Table for summary of recommendations.

Address for correspondence

SIGN Secretary
Royal College of Physicians
9 Queen Street
Edinburgh EH2 1JQ
UK

email: j.harlen@rcpe.ac.uk

http://www.show.scot.nhs.uk/sign/pdf/sign22.pdf

Summary of recommendations

	Grade
This guideline makes recommendations for management of the behavioural and psychological aspects of dementia, but excludes interventions in the management of cognitive aspects of dementia.	

Non-drug interventions

*On the basis of the available evidence and the problems associated with drug interventions, **non-drug interventions should always be considered along with drug options before treatment is started.***   C
Non-drug management strategies in the management of behavioural and psychological aspects of dementia include reality orientation, behavioural intervention, occupational activities, environmental modification, validation therapy, reminiscence and sensory stimulation.
A care plan should be made for each individual.

Neuroleptic drugs

Neuroleptics have been widely prescribed in the management of dementia, but evidence for their efficacy is limited.
***Patients should only be considered for treatment with neuroleptics if they have serious problems,** particularly psychotic symptoms, serious emotional distress or danger from behaviour disturbance.*   C
There is no clear evidence for the superiority of one neuroleptic drug over any other. The side-effect profiles differ.
***Low doses should be prescribed initially** with a slow and cautious increase if necessary: 'start low, go slow'.*   C
Treatment should normally be short term, and should be reviewed regularly.   B
***The prescriber must be aware of potential side-effects,** including akathisia and tardive dyskinesia. The routine use of anticholinergic medication is not indicated.*   C
***Care should be taken to identify Lewy body dementia** because of the increased risk of severe side effects.*   B

Use of other drugs

The evidence for the use of many described drug treatments for behaviour problems is not sufficient to make recommendations.
Marked and persistent depression in the presence of dementia may be treated with antidepressant medication.   B
Severe and persistent anxiety in the presence of dementia may require short-term anxiolytic treatment.   C
Severe and persistent insomnia in the presence of dementia may require short-term hypnotic treatment.   C
The issue of consent to treatment in the presence of dementia requires careful consideration, and use of the Mental Health (Scotland) Act 1984 may need to be considered.
Further research is required into the measurement of symptoms and the efficacy of interventions of all types.

Behavioral and Psychological Symptoms of Dementia: A Consensus Statement on Current Knowledge and Implications for Research and Treatment

Reference   Finkel SI, Cost e Silva J, Cohen GD, Miller S *et al* (1996) Behavioral and psychological signs and symptoms of dementia: a consensus statement on current knowledge and implications for research and treatment *International Psychogeriatrics* 8(Suppl 3): 497–500

Purpose

To describe current practice and research in behavioral and psychological symptoms of dementia.

Summary

This consensus statement arose out of a meeting organized by the International Psychogeriatric Association to discuss psychiatric symptoms and behavioral disturbances. One issue was resolving the nomenclature to be used to describe these various features. They were originally called non-cognitive features of dementia (Rosen *et al*, 1984; Burns *et al*, 1990), but that had the problem of being a rather negative description and also did not acknowledge the fact that many of them appeared to have their basis in cognitive dysfunction. An alternative description was neuropsychiatric features (Cummings *et al*, 1994) and under the descriptive term was BDD (Behavioral Disorders in Dementia) but as this did not capture many of the psychiatric components the term BPSSD (Behavioral and Psychological Signs and Symptoms of Dementia), which was shortened to BPSD (Behavioral and Psychological Symptoms of Dementia) was used. The term psychological was chosen rather than psychiatric because of the difficulties of stigmatization. One difficulty is that it perpetuates the notion of behavioral symptoms, which does not make phenomenological sense. The conclusions of the conference were:

1. The behavioral and psychological symptoms of dementia are integral elements of the disease process and are therefore a legitimate concern of healthcare providers worldwide.
2. These symptoms present severe problems to all those who interact with the patients, as well as to the patients themselves and to society and its health services.
3. Many of the behavioral and psychological symptoms of dementia are now amenable to treatment. Such treatment will reduce the suffering of the patients, the burden on the family, and the economic cost arising in connection with dementia.
4. Research now needs to address the following areas:
    *   development of cross-culturally applicable methods for the assessment of behavioral and psychological symptoms of dementia
    *   exploration of the relationship between behavioral and psychological symptoms of dementia with respect to the environments in which they occur and their underlying biological and psychological substrates.
    *   longitudinal evaluation of these symptoms
    *   determination of the frequency, underlying pathogenic mechanisms, and clinical and social impact on patient, family and society of the behavioral and psychological symptoms of dementia
    *   development of a well-defined profile of treatment methods with specific reference to different types of behavioral and psychological symptoms and their response to pharmacologic and non-pharmacologic interventions.

The Consenus Statement has recently been updated.

Finkel I, Burns A (2000) Behavioural and psychological symptoms of dementia: a clinical research update. *International psychogeriatrics* 12(suppl 1)

Additional references

Burns A, Jacoby R, Levy R (1990) Psychiatric phenomena in Alzheimer's disease. IV: Disorders of behaviour. *British Journal of Psychiatry* **157**: 86–94.

Cummings JL, Mega M, Gray K, Rosenberg-Thompson S, Carusi DA, Gornbein J (1994) The Neuropsychiatric Inventory: comprehensive assessment of psychopathology in dementia. *Neurology* 44: 2308–14.

Rosen WG, Mohs RC, Davis KL (1984) A new rating scale for Alzheimer's disease. *American Journal of Psychiatry* **141**: 1356–64.

Address for correspondence

International Psychogeriatric Association
550 Frontage Road
Suit 2820
Northfield, IL
USA

ipa@ipa-online.org

Bathing Persons with Dementia

Reference   University of Iowa Gerontological Nursing Interventions Research Center, Research Dissemination Core (1995). University of Iowa

Purpose

The aim of the guideline is to provide research-based recommendations for minimizing fear, agitation, combative behavior and the development of secondary behavioral symptoms during and/or after personal hygiene among patients with chronic dementing illnesses. These guidelines were developed using expert consensus based on all available data, documentation and published papers. The guidelines are intended for nurses and nurse practitioners.

Summary

Care must be individualized, and caregivers flexible, by focusing on the resident more than the tasks. It is important to understand the bathing history, using the resident's home as a focus (i.e. what would be reasonable if the person was at home). The method that is least distressing to the resident should be identified, and the time that the patient is unclothed should be minimized. The following specific recommendations are made: distraction and negotiation should be used instead of confrontation; the patient should be rewarded after the bathing experience with realistic praise. Finally, a list of strategies is provided to manage specific problems with bathing, e.g. when the patient does not want to go to the bathing area, when the resident resists getting into a tub or a shower, when the resident is cold, when the bathing is painful, when the resident is hollering and screaming, hitting, pinching or shoving, grabbing objects or people, and biting.

Address for correspondence

University of Iowa Gerontological Nursing Interventions Research Center
Research Dissemination Core
4118 Westlawn
Iowa City, IA 52242-1100
USA

Management of Decision-Making Capacity in Nursing Homes

Reference   Gerontological Nursing Interventions Research Center (1996, 1998) University of Iowa

MacLean DS (1996) Pilot study of impaired decision-making capacity in a nursing home. *Nursing Home Medicine* 4: 91–2

Purpose

The guideline provides direction for physicians and nursing facility interdisciplinary teams in assessing a nursing home resident's decision-making capacity.

Summary

Three levels or categories of decision-making capacity are defined:

- *Level 1* – Full decision-making capacity, where residents can make all decisions independently.
- *Level 2* – Limited decision-making capacity, where the resident has lost the ability to make one or more complex decisions independently, but still possesses at minimum the capacity to designate a Power of Attorney. For these residents, decision-making capacity may be sufficient for some decisions but not for others, and this may fluctuate over time.
- *Level 3* – Unable to make decisions, where the residents can make no legally significant decisions even with assistance. The demarcation of this low level of decision-making capacity is the inability to consistently recognize

family, and consequently the inability to designate a Power of Attorney. At this level, residents, while unable to make legally significant decisions, can still express simple preferences and choices such as food, clothing and daily routine.

According to the guideline, each newly admitted resident should be assessed for decision-making capacity and assigned a provisional assessment as either full, limited or unable to make decisions. During the initial 2-week stay, the interdisciplinary team should make further observations to determine decision-making capacity in four domains; civil, personal, financial and health care.

Address for correspondence

University of Iowa Gerontological Nursing Intervention Research Center
Department of Nursing – RDDC
University of Iowa Hospitals and Clinics
200 Hawkins Drive T 152 GH
Iowa City, IA 52242-1009
USA

Guidelines for Addressing Ethical and Legal Issues in Alzheimer's Disease Research: A Position Paper

Reference   High DM, Whitehouse PJ, Post SG, Berg L (1994) Guidelines for addressing ethical and legal issues in Alzheimer disease research: a position paper. *Alzheimer Disease and Associated Disorders* 8(Suppl 4): 66–74

Purpose

To summarize ethical and legal issues in Alzheimer's disease research.

Summary

Research with patients with Alzheimer's disease raises difficult ethical and legal questions because cognitively impaired people are involved. Increased participation in research by living subjects is occurring, and the point is made that researchers and sponsoring agencies need to provide for the rights and welfare of this special class of persons.

The publication represents a position paper developed by representatives of the 28 Alzheimer's disease centers in the USA. Six positions are described:

- Position 1: Equitable recruitment and selection of subjects
- Position 2: Respect for capacities of subjects
- Position 3: Role of families and proxy decision-makers in informed consent process
- Position 4: Enhancement of communication
- Position 5: Conflicts of interest
- Position 6: Risks and benefits.

Recommendations

1. Scientists and IRBs should ensure that recruitment, selection and enrolment of AD research subjects include ethnically and culturally diverse populations, women and minorities. Status of research subjects, such as preferring non-institutionalized, competent subjects over others, should be avoided as a means of selection. The use of homogeneous study populations must be justified on scientific grounds.

2. Research instruments and procedures, including diagnostic and cognitive testing, should be as free as possible from cultural biases. All outreach material and documents prepared for informed consent should be easily understood, taking into account level of education and literacy of subjects and their representatives.

3. Research protocols should specify the means for determining a subject's capacity for informed consent on a task-specific basis. Medical or neuropsychological assessment of AD is relevant to but not determinative of decision-making capacity.

4. Informed consent should be sought from competent AD subjects. For incompetent persons, informed consent should be sought from authorized surrogates together with assent from the AD subjects. When a subject's decision-making capacity is uncertain, effort should be made to obtain consent from both the subject and the surrogate.

5. Unless there is statutory or case law to the contrary, the presumptive authority of a family member to serve as a subject's representative should be followed without prerequisite appointment of a guardian or proxy with a durable power of attorney document.

6. Researchers should extend efforts to understand the communicative difficulties experienced by persons with AD and establish lines of communication that build mutual trust and cooperation.

7. Alzheimer's Disease Centers (ADCs) and researchers should encourage potential research subjects to make use of advance directives for research, including written and oral instructions and appointment of proxies.

8. Researchers should ensure that conflicts of interest are avoided when providing clinical care and recruiting patients for research protocols. They should disclose any significant financial and/or academic benefits that may accrue to investigators through the conduct of a particular research protocol.

9. Risks and potential harm to participants should always be minimized and benefits maximized. Caution should be exercised in claiming direct or peripheral benefits to subjects through AD research participation.

10. Research that involves potential risks and no direct benefit to subjects may be justified if the anticipated knowledge is vital and the research protocol is likely to generate such knowledge.

11. Attention should be given to understanding and interpreting degrees of risks to subjects and risk/benefit ratios. Type, magnitude and probability of risks should be considered in assessing and evaluating risks and benefits for AD research subjects.

12. ADCs and researchers should continue an ongoing dialog concerning the ethical and legal issues of AD research, recognizing that advances in research will produce new dilemmas.

Address for correspondence

Dr DM High
Alzheimer's Disease Research Center
101 Sanders-Brown Bldg
University of Kentucky
Lexington, KY 40536-0230
USA

Alzheimer's Disease and Related Dementias: Legal Issues in Care and Treatment

Reference   A report to Congress of the Advisory Panel on Alzheimer's Disease (1994)

www.alzheimers.org/pubs/legal94.html

Purpose

The Advisory Panel on Alzheimer's Disease was established with the mandate of assisting the Secretary of the Department of Health and Human Services and Council for Alzheimer's Disease in the identification of priorities in emerging issues with respect to Alzheimer's disease and related dementias, and the care of individuals with such disease and dementias.

Summary

This particular report focuses upon the legal issues arising in the context of Alzheimer's disease and has a number of categories:

1. The law and Alzheimer's disease
2. Autonomy and incapacity (voluntary and involuntary transfers of decision making)
3. Medical decision making
   - patient or presumed patient
   - advance directives
   - refusing medical treatment
   - treating in the absence of advance directives
   - federal involvement in medical decision making.

The Panel observes that: *this approach to the assessment of legal capacity in persons with AD poses a number of problems, including: (a) reliance on a medical evaluation in the absence of specifically identified tests; (b) adequacy of the diagnostic screens, if used; (c) the familiarity of the medical witness with current practices in diagnosis and evaluation of potential AD; (d) reliability of determinations made through an evaluation performed at a distinct point in time; and (e) absence of measures of judgment.*

Current best medical opinion holds that *clinical diagnoses of Alzheimer's disease should be established through careful clinical evaluation at several different points in time. That evaluation should include, but not be limited to: (a) cognitive screening instruments (such as the MMSE); (b) NINDS/ADRDA Alzheimer's screening criteria, including other neuropsychological assessment tools; and (c) measures of practical aspects of functioning such as occupational evaluations.* In addition, the assessment would be incomplete in the absence of historical evidence provided by the person in question or informed individuals, such as family and personal physician. The same determining procedures and methods should be employed across legal jurisdictions to bring greater uniformity to legal decision making about AD patients' capacity.

Alzheimer's disease's early feature of memory loss alone does not necessarily compromise a person's ability to make informed decisions or to express preferences; impairment of judgment arises in the course of the disease, not necessarily at its diagnosis. Courts should weigh this distinction carefully in competence determinations. Families and medical professionals too should be better informed about these distinctions.

The complexity of capacity determinations for persons with AD suggests that *greater uniformity in evaluations and the concomitant need for evaluations at multiple points in time are needed.* A person with AD may be competent for certain purposes at a given time, yet found incompetent for other purposes at the same time. For this reason, the Panel *recommends that courts consider implementing regularly scheduled reassessments of the legal capacity of persons with ADRD until such time as verbal and communication skills are irrevocably lost, thereby preserving autonomy in as many areas as possible for as long as possible.* The Panel concurs that when these skills are determined to be lost irrevocably, repeated determinations of decision-making ability are no longer necessary.

As the Panel found in its third report with respect to persons with AD, and as held as a key tenet of jurisprudence for the general population, individual autonomy and the right to make decisions should be granted primacy over the desires of others; these personal rights should also be safeguarded for as long as legally and medically possible. For these reasons, the Panel recommends that *the legal and medical communities work together to reach consensus on a specific set of tools through which the legal system may better be able to ascertain whether a person of uncertain cognitive status retains the legal capacity to enter into agreements of any sort, including the legal delegation of decision making. Standardization of these procedures nationwide is indicated,* since the incidence and prevalence of AD do not vary widely from state to state.

Greater education is needed about the utility and appropriateness of voluntary transfers of authority. Simple descriptions of what these mechanisms are and how they can be undertaken should be provided. Such information should be placed in the context of the nature of ADRD, its course, and its potential consequences on individual autonomy and decision making.

Because persons diagnosed in the early stages of AD often retain the ability to undertake voluntary transfers of decision making, health care professionals working with such persons should provide information about the mechanisms through which such voluntary delegations may be made. This is particularly important in states in which durable powers of attorney may be used to guide medical decisions at later stages of the disease process. From the perspective of the person with AD, the most important aspect of a voluntary transfer may be the early designation of a trusted, knowledgeable, specific surrogate decision-maker in the event of incapacity. *Professional societies, continuing education programs, and medical schools should help educate physicians about issues regarding voluntary transfers, since physicians often represent the most significant contact point for older Americans outside the family structure.* In this way, physicians may help assure patient autonomy for as long as possible, ensuring that patient desires are met even when decision-making capacity has been lost. The early establishment of a voluntary transfer can safeguard against the need for such determinations at the point of hospital admission, a time not ideal for patient-centered decision making.

The use of voluntary decision making should be encouraged.

Given the irreversible nature and destruction of cognitive ability inherent in AD, the Panel believes it critical that people express their wishes regarding care: (1) if they have received a tentative or confirming diagnosis of the disorder in its early stages; or (2) if there is any concern about potential future loss of cognitive ability.

In the Panel's opinion, AD today must be considered a terminal illness; end-stage AD is no less terminal than end-stage cancer or heart disease. The Panel understands that the uniform act on advance directives recently adopted by the National Commissioners of Uniform State law removes the requirement that end-stage disease be certified. However, until the model statute is adopted by each of the 50 states, the panel believes that determination of what constitutes 'end-stage' AD should be the province of the treating physician. The Panel further suggests that individual physicians, courts and families should be granted broad permission to establish when an advance directive of a person with ADRD should be honored.

The Panel believes that these same principles should guide the medical decision making that occurs in the care and treatment of Alzheimer's patients. To that end, and as stated earlier in this paper, the Panel recommends that *given the nature and destruction of cognitive ability inherent in AD, people should be encouraged to express their wishes regarding care through the use of advance directives. Such directives are warranted whether the individual is at risk of AD, has received a tentative or confirming diagnosis of the disorder, or if there is any concern about potential loss of cognitive ability in the future.*

Greater research is warranted regarding the stability of treatment preferences over time.

By suggesting the use of advance directives, the Panel is also arguing for *further basic and clinical research that may lead to the detection of AD in its very earliest stages*, before questions that could cloud the validity of an advance directive arise, such as issues of capacity or cognitive status.

Yet, even with an advance directive in place, its utility has been limited by the laws governing such documents. Most often, a right to refuse treatment (contained in an advance directive) is limited to cases of terminal illness. Unfortunately, neither case history nor general practice of medicine or law is clear regarding precisely how AD falls within that definition. In the Panel's view, until such time as the uniform act on advance directives is enacted in each state, *both those rendering treatment of AD patients and those defining status governing the right to refuse treatment today must consider AD to be a terminal illness. End-stage AD should be treated in the same way as end-stage heart disease or cancer; advance directives should be honored based on the treating physician's determination that the illness has reached its final stage.* As observed in its previous reports, the Panel recognizes the difficulties inherent in linking such policy principles to clinical care or personal decisions by individual patients and families. Nonetheless, the issue remains one of values, and those of the individual with AD should remain paramount in the medical and legal decision-making processes.

Conclusion

This report represents the culmination of several years of Advisory Panel deliberations regarding legal issues affecting the care and treatment of people with Alzheimer's disease. The issues are complex, ranging from questions of autonomy and capacity to medical treatment and the right to refuse that treatment. The lengthy trajectory of AD further complicates how decisions regarding the legal rights of a person with AD are to be protected, and also how that person's safety is to be maintained. The Panel's Third Report emphasized the role of values in the care and treatment of persons with AD. Values form an overarching theme in this report as well, including the values implied in law and statute, the values inherent in the voluntary transfer of decision making, the values held by formal and informal caregivers, and the values contained in advance directives.

The legal implications of Alzheimer's disease have not been clarified in case law to date. However, as the number of persons with AD rises, the need for more reasoned and medically sound mechanisms to determine issues of capacity and stage of illness is heightened. To that end, the Panel has made a host of recommendations regarding legal capacity and medical decision making in AD care and treatment:

1. Medical and legal determinations of cognitive ability and judgment are not synonymous. Courts should

weigh this distinction in competence determinations; families and medical professionals should be better informed of the differences.

2. Greater uniformity in medical evaluations and the conduct of evaluations at different points in time can help ensure that the autonomy of a person with AD may be maintained for as long as possible.

3. The legal and medical communities should work together to reach consensus on specific nationally applicable tools through which the legal system may be able to ascertain whether a person of uncertain cognitive status retains the legal capacity to make his or her own decisions.

4. The use and appropriateness of voluntary transfers of authority should be the subject of education for older persons and their families, through not only ADRD-related organizations, but also programs working with older Americans in general, whether at the Federal, state or local levels. Health professionals, too, should be educated about such mechanisms, and should provide information about them to their patients or clients. Professional societies, continuing education programs and medical schools can be helpful in this effort.

5. The use of advance directives should be encouraged for those at risk of or those diagnosed with AD. Through improved methods of early detection of AD, the timely issuance of such directives can be facilitated. Until such time as the model uniform act on advance directives is adopted by each of the states, the use of advance directives, however, must be accompanied by acceptance of the Panel's view that there is such a concept as 'end-stage' AD and that the trajectory of AD today is no different from that of a patient diagnosed with incurable heart disease or cancer.

The Panel believes that enactment of the recommendations contained in this report will be beneficial not only to large numbers of ADRD patients and their families, but also to the wider community. It calls upon those in the medical and legal professions to begin to grapple with the legal issues surrounding Alzheimer's disease from the perspective of the patient and family, urging greater education of older Americans and caregivers about legal mechanisms available to preserve individual autonomy in the event of lost cognitive capacity due to ADRD.

Ethical Guidelines of the Alzheimer Society of Canada

Reference   Fisk JD, Sadovnick AD, Cohen CA, Gauthier S, Dossetor J, Eberhart A and Le Duc L (1998) Ethical guidelines of the Alzheimer Society of Canada. *Canadian Journal of Neuroscience* 25: 242–8

Purpose

To facilitate the discussion of the ethics of care of people with Alzheimer's disease. The guidelines were developed using an extensive nationwide consultation process and built on the 'Fairhill Guidelines'. Initial draft guidelines were presented in April 1996 at an Annual Conference of The Alzheimer Society of Canada. The initial draft guidelines were distributed across Canada via the Alzheimer Society provincial organizations to obtain feedback. The guidelines and feedback were discussed at a workshop in December 1996, and this resulted in the final draft of the guidelines that were approved by the Board of Directors in February 1997.

Summary

The guidelines deal with the following issues: communicating the diagnosis; driving; respect in individual choice; quality of life; participation in research; genetic testing; the use of restraints; end of life care.

Communicating the diagnosis: Affected individuals and their families should be informed about the diagnosis and directed to appropriate support services in a sensitive manner.

Driving: Throughout the course of the disease the person's driving ability needs to be monitored collaboratively by family members, physicians and/or other health care professionals. It is vital that all those involved in this process of monitoring communicate with one another. When the person's driving is recognized as dangerous, automobile access must be removed immediately.

Respecting individual choice: While still capable, the individual should be given choices and the opportunity to make decisions. Ideally the individual has planned the time when she or he can no longer make decisions, and has identified another individual who will take his or her prior wishes into consideration.

Quality of life: Individuals with Alzheimer's disease are able to find pleasure and experience satisfaction. The disease does not remove the ability to appreciate and respond, or the ability to experience feelings such as anger, fear, joy, love or sadness.

Participation in research: Individuals with Alzheimer's disease at any stage should have the opportunity to participate in research and their desires should be primary when considering participation in research. When the individual is no longer able to provide informed consent and a substitute decision maker makes the decision regarding participation, the research team has an obligation to ensure that the decision has been guided by the individual's wishes and/or that it has been made with the individual's best interest in mind. The research team must maintain an ongoing dialogue with the individual, his or her family and care providers. Participation of individuals with Alzheimer's disease in research often places demands on their family and care providers. All such individuals should be involved in the consent process and in the assessment of the consequences of participation.

Genetic testing: At this point in time, for the vast majority of individuals, there is no test, genetic or non-genetic, to determine if a specific unaffected individual will develop Alzheimer's disease. Even for the very rare individual for whom it is possible to predict the future development of Alzheimer's disease based on genetic status, the decision to know or not to know is a personal one which must be made in a setting that allows for informed consent, genetic and psychological counselling, and confidentiality.

Use of restraints: The guidelines recommend that no restraints be used. The inappropriate use of restraints results in the individual with Alzheimer's disease losing those skills and ability needed for daily activities. Once those skills and abilities have been lost, they are unlikely to be regained. Should there be special reasons for considering the use of restraints, the risks and benefits to the individual and those around them must be weighed. If the use of restraints can be justified, they must be used for a limited time only, and must be accompanied by well-defined goals and very close monitoring.

End of life care: Respect for the individual's expressed wishes and interest should guide all end-of-life care decisions. In the transition from life to death, the ultimate goal of care should be to provide comfort and dignity to the person, towards achieving what the individual considers to be a 'good death'. What defines a good death differs from individual to individual. In planning a good death, individuals should take into consideration cultural, religious, spiritual and family values.

Address for correspondence

John D Fisk
Alzheimer Society of Canada
20 Eglinton Ave West, Suite 1200
Toronto, Ontario
M4R 1K8
Canada

Fairhill Guidelines on Ethics of the Care of People with Alzheimer's Disease – a Clinical Summary

Reference   Post SG, Whitehouse PJ, Center for Biomedical Ethics, Case Western Reserve University and the Alzheimer's Association (1995) Fairhill guidelines on ethics of the care of people with Alzheimer's disease: a clinical summary. *Journal of the American Geriatric Society* 43: 1423–9

Purpose

These guidelines were developed through focus meetings with mild Alzheimer's patients' family carers, who met on a monthly basis over a period of 9 months. They deal with such issues as truth-telling and diagnosis, driving privileges, respecting choice, the level of behavioral control, issues with death and dying, quality of life and treatment decisions. These guidelines are important because they take into consideration the voice of people with mild dementia.

Summary

Truth telling and diagnosis: Doctors should inform affected patients and their families about the diagnosis of Alzheimer's disease. The disclosure of the diagnosis brings certain responsibilities, including directing the individual and the family to appropriate resources, and the development of an appropriate care plan.

Driving privileges: The diagnosis of Alzheimer's disease is not sufficient reason to take away driving privileges. The duty to prevent driving should not be applied too early without an individualized risk assessment demonstrating impairment of driving ability. Restrictions in driving and self-termination of driving should be negotiated between the patient and the physician. Driving privileges should not be revoked without identifying alternative ways of getting around. A gradual, caring, negotiated approach to restrictions is the best way forward. This protects privileges and freedom as much as possible, while making efforts to substitute other activities for the ones that are lost.

Respecting choice: The development of Alzheimer's disease does not mean loss of capacity in all areas. People with dementia should be allowed to exercise their remaining capacity for specific tasks and choices as much as possible. Task-specific capacity cannot be determined solely on the basis of cognitive test scores. There must be considered questioning and discussion to examine the level of understanding and reasoning capacity for the specific task under scrutiny.

Dilemmas of behavioral control: The dangers and difficulties of physical restraints are summarized. Strangulation, medical ailments caused by immobility and increased agitation are among the harms caused by physical restraints. While the value of patient safety is very important, it does not justify involuntary restraint and the indignity of being tied down, except perhaps on a very temporary basis in extreme circumstances such as delirium. Behavioral controlling drugs should be used cautiously and for specified purposes. The dangers of polypharmacy and over-medication are highlighted, and when drugs are used they should be used at low doses.

Issues of death and dying: Issues of death and dying are not discussed sufficiently with patients and their carers. A physician who provides continuing care for people with dementia should initiate discussion with patients and their family regarding the use of aggressive measures to prolong life. Conflicts and disagreements between affected individuals and their families can best be avoided and resolved through early and continuing communication. Empowerment of individual choice will allow family members to deal with unforeseen situations through the methods of a Will, and Enduring Power of Attorney.

Quality of life and treatment decisions: It can be very difficult to measure quality of life in people with dementia. Formal carers and family members often assess the quality of life in the Alzheimer's individual more negatively than is justified. It would appear that the majority of older nursing home residents would only want comfort care and palliation in the event of advanced Alzheimer's disease. The quality of life in a nursing home requires a commitment to the autonomy of individuals and respect for their treatment refusals. An example of maintaining caloric intake in advanced dementia is cited. When individuals have profound and terminal dementia they are often provided with artificial feeding, although clinical evidence is available which indicates that foregoing foods and nutrition in end-stage illness does not cause suffering, while providing nutrition artificially can cause unpleasant side effects such as bloating and aspiration pneumonia.

Conclusions

There are a range of ethical concerns that must be considered as society ages and as Alzheimer's disease becomes more prevalent. One of the most urgent concerns for medical ethics and society is the fact that there is decline of the mind within a still viable body. The guidelines emphasize that emotional and relational wellbeing can be enhanced despite dementia, as long as human dignity is respected.

Address for correspondence

Stephen G Post PhD
Center for Biomedical Ethics
Great Western Reserve University School of Medicine
Room T 402, 10900 Euclid Ave
Cleveland, OH 44106-497, USA

Ethical Issues in the Management of the Demented Patient

Reference   The American Academy of Neurology Ethics and Humanities Subcommittee (1996) *Neurology* **46:** 1180–3

Purpose

To address how ethical considerations influence ideal patient management (not intended to represent clinical practice guidelines).

Summary

Six areas are considered:

1. Patient–physician relationship
2. Advance directives for medical care
3. Proxy decision making
4. Family of the demented patient
5. Restraining the demented patient
6. Palliative care and withholding and withdrawing life-sustaining treatment.

1. *Patient–physician relationship.* The principles should emphasize the priority of care over cure by
   - paying careful attention to the seemingly minor but personally important details of the patient's daily life, e.g. nutrition, bowel function, sleep, safety, agitation and incontinence
   - identifying and treating depression in elderly people who may present as pseudodementia
   - limiting and monitoring the number and doses of different medications.
   - rigorous treatment of coexisting medical problems, e.g. diabetes, hypertension, lung disease
   - correcting sensory deficits
   - encouraging patients to stop smoking and drinking
   - encouraging appropriate nutrition and vitamin supplementation if necessary
   - providing continuity of care.
2. *Advanced directives for medical care.* It is stated that neurologists should urge all patients, including those with the early stages of dementia, to complete advance directives for medical care and to educate them about the potential adverse consequences of not doing so. Where the patient is incompetent, the consent of an appropriate proxy decision-maker is necessary for all non-emergency tests and treatments.
3. *Proxy decision making.* Advance directives should be followed as faithfully as is possible and reasonable. In their absence, an appropriate proxy decision-maker should be identified to make health care decisions for the patient.
4. *The family of the demented patient.* It is desirable for neurologists to maximize the success of the home caregiver of the demented patient, thereby permitting the demented patient more time to live at home, by: (a) education; (b) identification and minimization of caregiver stress; (c) prevention of caregiver burden.
5. *Restraining demented patients.* Guidelines to be observed in the ordering of mechanical or pharmacological restraints are: (a) they should be ordered when they contribute to the safety of the patient or others and not just as a convenience; (b) they should not be routinely ordered; (c) the perceived need for restraint should trigger a medical investigation for the precise reason for them; (d) restraints should be ordered with informed consent by the patient or appropriate proxy decision-maker; (e) the least restrictive device should be used; (f) pharmacological restraints should be prescribed with the proper agent in the lowest dose possible; (g) all orders for restraint should be reassessed frequently.
6. *Palliative care and withholding and withdrawing life-sustaining treatment.* Palliative care refers to the class of orders of medical and nursing treatment that is intended to maximize patient comfort but not necessarily extend life – palliative care provides symptomatic treatment for disorders that produce patient discomfort, but omits curative treatment for those disorders that do not result in patient discomfort even if the patient may die sooner as a result of the lack of curative treatment. Palliative care is not to cause death but rather to permit it in as gentle, comfortable and pain-free a fashion as possible. A palliative care plan should include oxygen, cleared airways, morphine for dyspnea, atropine for comfortable secretions, morphine for pain, antipyretics for fever, mouth care, bathing, grooming, skin care, bowel and bladder care, positioning, and a passive range of motion exercises. Cardiopulmonary resuscitation attempts are not performed, and hospital admissions and surgeries are avoided unless it is likely that they will improve patient comfort. Oral hydration and nutrition are offered, assisted and encouraged, but hydration and nutrition are not provided by artificial enteral or parenteral means unless they contribute to patient comfort or are chosen by the patient or proxy.

Address for correspondence

Dr JL Bernat
Neurology Section
Dartmouth-Hitchcock Medical Center
Lebanon, NH 03756, USA

At-a-Glance Guide to the Current Medical Standards of Fitness to Drive

Reference   Drivers Medical Unit, DVLA Swansea UK (1999)

Purpose

To summarize the medical guidelines of fitness to drive. The UK Secretary of State for Transport, the Environment and the Regions has the responsibility, via his medical advisors, for the Drivers' Medical Unit, DVLA to ensure that all license holders are fit to drive.

Summary

It is the duty of the license holder or applicant to notify DVLA of any medical condition which may affect safe driving. There are some circumstances in which the licensee cannot or will not do this. Under these circumstances the General Medical Council has issued clear guidelines. These are:

1. The DVLA is legally responsible for deciding if a person is medically unfit to drive. They need to know when driving license holders have a condition which now or in the future may affect their safety as a driver.
2. Therefore, where patients have such conditions, you should
   - make sure that the patients understand that the condition may impair their ability to drive. If a patient is incapable of understanding this advice, for example because of dementia, you should inform the DVLA immediately
   - explain to patients that they have a legal duty to inform the DVLA about the condition.
3. If the patients refuse to accept the diagnosis or the effect of the condition on their ability to drive, you can suggest that the patients seek a second opinion, and make appropriate arrangements for the patients to do so. You should advise patients not to drive until the second opinion has been obtained.
4. If patients continue to drive when they are not fit to do so, you should make every reasonable effort to persuade them to stop. This may include telling their next of kin.
5. If you do not manage to persuade patients to stop driving, or you are given or find evidence that a patient is continuing to drive contrary to advice, you should

disclose relevant medical information immediately, in confidence, to the medical advisor at DVLA.

6. Before giving information to the DVLA, you should inform the patient of your decision to do so. Once the DVLA has been informed, you should also write to the patient, to confirm that a disclosure has been made.

Dementia or any organic brain syndrome

DVLA must be notified as soon as diagnosis is made. It is extremely difficult to assess driving ability in those with dementia. Those who have poor short-term memory, disorientation, lack of insight and judgment are almost certainly not fit to drive. The variable presentations and rates of progression are acknowledged. Disorders of attention will also cause impairment. A decision regarding fitness to drive is usually based on medical reports. In early dementia, when sufficient skills are retained and progression is slow, a licence may be issued subject to annual review. A formal driving assessment may be necessary.

Elderly drivers

Age is no bar to holding a license. DVLA require confirmation at age 70 that no medical disability is present; thereafter a 3-year license is issued subject to satisfactory completion of medical questions on the application form. Notwithstanding, as ageing progresses, a driver or his/her relative(s) may be aware that the combination of progressive loss of memory, impairment in concentration and reaction time with possible loss of confidence, suggest consideration be given to ceasing driving. Physical frailty is not *per se* a bar to the holding of a license.

Address for correspondence

Driver and Vehicle Licensing Agency
Drivers Medical Unit
Longview Road
Swansea SA99 1DA
UK

Practice Parameter: Risk of Driving and Alzheimer's Disease (An Evidence-Based Review)

Reference   Dubinsky RM, Stein AC, Lyons K (2000) Practice parameter: risk of driving and Alzheimer's disease (an evidence-based review) Report of the Quality Standards Subcommittee of the American Academy of Neurology. *Neurology* 54: 2205–11

Purpose

To develop practice parameters regarding driving and Alzheimer's disease, based on a systematic review of the literature and a summary.

Summary

Driving was found to be mildly impaired in those drivers with probable AD at a severity of clinical dementia rating (CDR). This impairment was no greater than that tolerated in other segments of the driving population (e.g. drivers age 16–21 and those driving under the influence of alcohol at a blood alcohol concentration <0.08%). Drivers with AD at a severity of CDR 1 were found to pose significant traffic safety problems, both from crashes and from driving performance measurements.

Statement of the evidence

In patients with AD who continue to drive, there is clear evidence based on one Class I (Hunt *et al*) and several Class II studies (see Appendix 1) that there is an increased risk of crashes compared to age-matched controls. The relative risk of crashes for drivers with AD of CDR stage 1.0 is greater than our society tolerates for any group of drivers. Drivers with AD at CDR stage 0.5 have an increased risk of accidents similar to that accepted by society for 16–19-year-old drivers and for those drivers intoxicated with alcohol at a blood alcohol concentration <0.08%. This increased risk is based upon crash statistics, performance studies of drivers with AD, and testing of components of the driving task. Almost all of the reports that met the inclusion or exclusion criteria of our analysis found that cognitively impaired drivers fared worse than controls. However, most of the accident statistics research on drivers with AD has not taken driving exposure into account, has not relied on blinded evaluators, and has not included an adequate sample size. It is also difficult to compare the severity of dementia across studies; therefore whether the drivers with AD in most of the studies we reviewed really had an accident rate greater than society tolerates in younger drivers (aged 16–19) is moot. However, there is no doubt that the accident rate in the group with dementia is high. As to the relationship of degree of dementia to the accident rate, the CDR stages are based upon many levels of functioning of a patient with AD. Unfortunately, conversion of other scales to an equivalent of CDR stage 0.5 requires the combining of several dissimilar groups: mild cognitive impairment, questionable AD, and mild AD. Difficulties were also encountered converting the dissimilar scales used in these studies to an equivalent CDR. Given these difficulties, recommendations are made using the criteria for strength of evidence (Appendix 2). The published evidence on driving performance in those with AD supports the following recommendations. Decisions regarding license restrictions for drivers with AD must always be made in compliance with appropriate state laws and in consultation with the individual patient.

1. Patients and their families should be told that patients with AD with a severity of CDR 2 or greater have a substantially increased accident rate and driving performance errors, and therefore should not drive an automobile (Standard).

2. Patients and their families should be told that patients with possible AD with a severity of CDR 0.5 pose a significant traffic safety problem when compared to other elderly drivers. Referral of the patient for a driving performance evaluation by a qualified examiner should be considered (Guideline). Because of the high likelihood of progression to a severity of CDR 1 within a few years, clinicians should reassess dementia severity and appropriateness of continued driving every 6 months (Standard)

Appendix 1: Classes of evidence

- *Class I:* Must have all the following: (a) prospective study of well-defined cohorts that includes a description of the nature of the population, the inclusion or exclusion criteria, demographic characteristics (such as age, sex) and commonly used staging of dementia severity; (b) the sample size must be adequate with enough statistical power to justify the conclusions or for identification of subgroups for whom testing does or does not yield significant information; (c) the interpretation of evaluations performed must be done blinded to subject status; (d) the methodology used for evaluations must be adequate.
- *Class II:* (a) a retrospective study of a well-defined cohort which otherwise meets criteria for Class Ia, Ib and Id; (b) a prospective or retrospective study which lacks any of the following: adequate sample size, a well-defined

control group, adequate methodology, blinding of evaluators, a description of the inclusion or exclusion criteria, and information such as age, sex and commonly used staging of dementia severity.

- *Class III:* may have either a, b or c: (a) criteria of a Class II article published in a non-peer-reviewed format; (b) a small cohort or case report; (c) evidence from expert opinion or consensus.

Appendix 2: Levels of recommendations
Recommendation (level of evidence):

- *Standard:* A principle for patient management that reflects a high degree of clinical certainty (usually this requires Class I evidence that directly addresses the clinical questions, or overwhelming Class II evidence when circumstances preclude randomized clinical trials.
- *Guideline:* A recommendation for patient management

for which the clinical utility is uncertain (inconclusive or conflicting evidence or opinion).
- *Practice advisory:* A practice recommendation for emerging or newly approved therapies or technologies based on evidence for at least one Class I study. The evidence may demonstrate only a modest statistical effect or limited (partial) clinical response, or significant cost–benefit questions may exist. Substantial (or potential) disagreement among practitioners or between payers and practitioners may exist.

Address for correspondence
Wendy Edlund
The Quality Standards Subcommittee
American Academy of Neurology
1080 Montreal Avenue
St Paul, MN 55116
USA

Dementia and Driving: An Attempt at Consensus

Reference Lundberg C, Johannsson K, Ball K *et al* (1997) Dementia and driving: an attempt at consensus. *Alzheimer Disease and Associated Disorders* 11: 28–37

Purpose

The consensus statement is aimed at providing primary care physicians with practical advice concerning the assessment of cognitive status in relation to driving.

Summary

The consensus is based on a review of existing research, and the consensus was reached on the statement that a diagnosis of moderate to severe dementia precludes driving and that certain individuals with mild dementia should be considered for a specialized assessment of their driving competence.

Guidelines for the family physician

It is of great importance that the issue of driving be handled in a sensitive and thoughtful manner, taking into account the needs of the patient and family, access to alternative transportation, and so on. If the physician comes to the conclusion that the patient is too impaired to continue driving, it should be made clear to the patient and accompanying family members. This decision should be documented in the medical record and given to the patient in writing (as well as to the caregiver or responsible party when warranted).

The consensus group agreed that documentation of a diagnosis of moderate to severe dementia (established by a comprehensive assessment of cognitive and functional abilities and usually corresponding to a rating of 2 or 3 on the Clinical Dementia Rating Scale) can, in itself, be considered sufficient to warrant a recommendation of immediate cessation of driving. In a situation where the cognitive impairment is mild, the demented patient whose functional level is stable in terms of sensory functions, perception, cognition and other functions related to traffic safety can be followed up at periodic intervals. However, when such a patient shows signs of functional deterioration, manifest as a breakdown of ADL or IADL skills, especially when combined with other impairments (e.g. borderline visual acuity or poor motor function), a thorough assessment of driving and driving-related abilities should be carried out. There was no consensus concerning the use of rating scores on the MMSE as elements of the decision-making process. A summary of the different approaches to this matter is found in the addendum to the present consensus document.

The group of individuals with cognitive impairment who do not have a formal diagnosis is extremely heterogeneous, and it is of great importance to determine the causes of the impairment. There is clinical evidence that driving fitness may often be compromised in patients who have been assessed at a dementia clinic but who have not been diagnosed with a dementing disease. For this group, however, cessation of driving should not be advised without a specialized assessment investigating the reasons for the patient's cognitive impairment, as well as gathering information upon which to base a decision concerning future driving. As long as the mildly impaired non-demented person has a stable and acceptable functional level and no evidence of driving impairment, a periodic follow-up is sufficient.

In all cases where a cognitively impaired patient (with or without a diagnosis of dementia) has been considered sufficiently safe to drive, whether or not the decision is based on a specialized assessment, the physician must follow up the case at regular intervals. The length of these intervals will depend on the aetiology and rate of progression of the cognitive impairment. Clinical experience shows that an existing legal obligation for physicians to instruct their patients about driving greatly facilitates discussions with patients and their families. The physician should make the patient and family aware of the increased risk of crashes among cognitively impaired individuals and, whenever possible, advise them about possible adaptive driving strategies to maximize the period during which the patient can safely drive. Examples of such strategies are avoiding unfamiliar surroundings, driving only during the day, and keeping longer distances between themselves and the cars ahead. The aim is a graduated exit from driving rather than an abrupt cessation. The process of graduated exit would also imply a gradual adaptation to alternative transportation.

Whenever the physician is concerned about the patient's driving but is uncertain about the extent of the patient's cognitive impairment and its influence on driving ability, he or she should refer the patient for more specialized assessment. If the driving patient constitutes an imminent danger to himself or others, the physician should report the patient to the authorities. However, the mandatory reporting of such cases in Sweden today does not appear to have the favour of medical practitioners, since so few drivers are reported per year. There is a concern that the relationship between patient and doctor might be endangered by consistent mandatory reporting, in particular, if a diagnosis of dementia in itself automatically leads to a revocation of the driving license. The risk of being brought to the attention of the authorities in such cases might make patients reluctant to seek assessment for medical problems in general and cognitive disorders in particular, and thus they may not benefit from the support provided by the medical services or, in some cases, may not be treated for a reversible condition.

Additional reference

Johannsson K, Lundberg C (1997) The 1994 international consensus conference on dementia and driving: a brief report. *Alzheimer Disease and Associated Disorders* 11(Suppl 1): 62–9

Address for correspondence

C Lundberg
Traffic Medicine Center
Division of Geriatric Medicine
Karolinska Institutet
Huddinge University Hospital
B84, S-141 86 Huddinge
Sweden

Fitness to Drive and Cognition

Reference   British Psychological Society (2001)

Purpose

A report produced by the Multidisciplinary Working Party on Acquired Neuropsychological Deficits and Fitness to Drive of the British Psychological Society. The document concerns the assessment of drivers with neuropsychological deficits acquired as a consequence of neurological conditions such as traumatic brain injury, stroke and dementia.

Summary

The document contains the following sections:

1. **Driving, health and the law**
Summarises current UK notification procedures and professional responsibilities

2. **The extent of the problem – Neurological impairments and driving**
Discusses changes in the complexity of the driving task, the impact of demographic changes, and the impact of specific neurological conditions upon road safety. Assessment of fitness to drive is complex and correlates poorly with clinical judgements. Similarly, the extent of the risk posed by drivers with dementia and other neurological conditions is hard to estimate.

3. **Current approaches to assessing driving competence**
Three aspects of assessment are discussed:
   i)   behavioural/psychological skills underlying normal driving performance and their assessment
   ii) neuropsychological assessment of fitness to drive
   iii) practical assessment of driving ability; including the use of assessment under road and simulated driving conditions and the role of Mobility Centres in this process.

4. **Future research needs and implications for clinical practice**
This includes developing more appropriate methods of screening and more detailed assessment, and the need to address specific questions, for example a better understanding of the skills involved in 'normal' driving and how these relate to clinical populations.

An appendix contains a summary of research on driving and neuropsychological tests.

In conclusion, the report calls for improved screening of licence holders with potential neuropsychological impairments. Such screening could be incorporated within standard clinical procedures. A three-stage process for assessment is suggested, starting with initial brief screening by relevant health workers, through a secondary more elaborate psychological/neuropsychological assessment for cases of intermediate complexity, to specialist assessment by Mobility Centres. The report also calls for the UK Department of Health to take a more active role on the issue of mobility for patients with neurological conditions.

Address for correspondence

British Psychological Society
St Andrews House
48 Princess Road East
Leicester
LE1 7DR
UK

Making Decisions

Reference   Lord Chancellor's Department (1999)

Purpose
Plans to reform the law on making decisions on behalf of mentally incapacitated adults.

Summary
This document follows detailed consideration of the responses to the 1997 consultation paper 'Who Decides' (www.open.gov.uk/lcd/menincap/ch1.htm), where 4000 responses were received from a wide variety of individuals. Two previous documents of relevance are the *Law Commission Report No 231 on Mental Incapacity* published by the Law Commission in 1995, and the *Law Commission Report (Consultation Paper 129) Mentally Incapacitated Adults and Decision Making: Medical Treatment and Research*.

The key aspects of 'Making Decisions' were as follows.

Definition of incapacity
The Government has decided new laws are needed to set out a new test of capacity and a new statutory definition of incapacity, based on definitions proposed by the Law Commission.

There will be a statutory presumption against lack of capacity; it will be assumed that people can make their own decisions unless it is proved they are unable to do so. This follows the principle that intervention into peoples' lives should be kept to the minimum.

Best interests
There will also be statutory guidance on how the best interest of mentally incapacitated people should be determined, based on the fullest possible participation of the individuals concerned, the views of those who care for them, and the prospects of their recovering mental capacity.

General authority
Future legislation will provide carers with a general authority to act reasonably for the personal welfare or health care of a mentally incapacitated person – a legal context for all the day-to-day decisions that have to be made, such as paying bills, giving medication, helping with dressing or feeding. When people act in accordance with this general authority, they will be protected from civil liability.

The general authority will not allow a carer access to savings belonging to an incapacitated person held in a bank or other financial institution, or give any authority in areas such as consent to marriage, sexual relations, adoption, divorce, parental responsibilities or voting rights.

Legislation, or a code of practice, will clarify the legal position on the liability for paying bills of someone who arranges goods or services for a mentally incapacitated person.

Lord Irvine said:

> this is an important and sensitive area of social policy which affects the daily lives of many people – the mentally incapacitated and those who care for them and make decisions for them and act on their behalf.
>
> The present law offers little protection to someone who is unable to make decisions or to the carer whose actions would have little or no legal basis. The Government has set out to provide an understandable framework in which the interests of the mentally incapacitated are protected and in which carers can act with confidence.

Continuing Power of Attorney
The Government also intends to improve the arrangements which people can make in case they become mentally incapacitated in future.

At present, an Enduring Power of Attorney allows people to nominate someone else to look after their financial affairs should they ever become unable to do so themselves. The Government intends to introduce a wider Continuing Power of Attorney to allow people to delegate decision making on health care and personal welfare, as well as financial matters, in case they become unable to make these decisions themselves.

The legislation will allow people to appoint more than one attorney, and will include a range of safeguards as to how Continuing Powers of Attorney are conducted.

Court of Protection
The Government has also decided that there will be a new single court jurisdiction, which will deal with all areas of decision making for adults without mental capacity. The new Court of Protection will be able to make decisions on behalf of people who cannot do so for themselves, and make declarations about mental capacity. It will also be able

to appoint a manager to make some decisions on a mentally incapacitated person's behalf.

The new Court will be led by a designated senior judge. High Court, Circuit and District judges will be assigned to the court, and health care, welfare and disputed financial cases involving the mentally incapacitated will be dealt with in the Regions as well as in London.

Living wills

In the light of responses to consultation, the Government has decided that a number of issues raised in *Who Decides?* should not be taken forward at this time.

These include advance statements about health care – sometimes called living wills – in which people set out the medical treatment they would or would not wish to receive should they ever become mentally incapacitated. In this area, consultation showed widely differing views held with deep conviction.

The Government Report sets out a clear statement of the present legal position on living wills. It confirms that guidance contained in case law, together with the Code of Practice published by the British Medical Association, provide sufficient clarity and flexibility to enable the validity of advance statements to be decided on a case by case basis. The government will keep the subject under consideration in the light of medical and legal developments.

Address for correspondence

Lord Chancellor's Department
Selborne House
54–60 Victoria Street
London SW1E 6QW
UK

www.open.gov.uk

Reference Guide to Consent for Examination and Treatment

Reference: UK Department of Health (2001)
             www.doh.gov.uk/consent

When do health professionals need consent from patients?

1. Before you examine, treat or care for competent adult patients you must obtain their consent.

2. Adults are always assumed to be competent unless demonstrated otherwise. If you have doubts about their competence, the question to ask is: "can this patient understand and weigh up the information needed to make this decision?" Unexpected decisions do not prove the patient is incompetent, but may indicate a need for further information or explanation.

3. Patients may be competent to make some health care decisions, even if they are not competent to make others.

4. Giving and obtaining consent is usually a process, not a one-off event. Patients can change their minds and withdraw consent at any time. If there is any doubt, you should always check that the patient still consents to your caring for or treating them.

Can children consent for themselves?

5. Before examining, treating or caring for a child, you must also seek consent. Young people aged 16 and 17 are presumed to have the competence to give consent for themselves. Younger children who understand fully what is involved in the proposed procedure can also give consent (although their parents will ideally be involved). In other cases, someone with parental responsibility must give consent on the child's behalf, unless they cannot be reached in an emergency. If a competent child consents to treatment, a parent **cannot** over-ride that consent. Legally, a parent can consent if a competent child refuses, but it is likely that taking such a serious step will be rare.

Who is the right person to seek consent?

6. It is always best for the person actually treating the patient to seek the patient's consent. however, you may seek consent on behalf of colleagues if you are capable of performing the procedure in question, or if you have been specially trained to seek consent for that procedure.

What information should be provided?

7. Patients need sufficient information before they can decide whether to give their consent: for example information about the benefits and risks of the proposed treatment, and alternative treatments. If the patient is not offered as much information as they reasonably need to make their decision, and in a form they can understand, their consent may not be valid.

Is the patient's consent voluntary?

8. Consent must be given voluntarily: not under any form of duress or undue influence from health professionals, family or friends.

Does it matter how the patient gives consent?

9. No: consent can be written, oral or non-verbal. A signature on a consent form does not itself prove the consent is valid – the point of the form is to record the patient's decision, and also increasingly the discussions that have taken place. Your Trust or organisation may have a policy setting out when you need to obtain written consent.

Refusals of treatment

10. Competent adult patients are entitled to refuse treatment, even where it would clearly benefit their health. The only exception to this rule is where the treatment is for a mental disorder and the patient is detained under the *Mental Health Act 1983*. A competent pregnant woman may refuse any treatment, even if this would be detrimental to the fetus.

Adults who are not competent to give consent

11. **No-one** can give consent on behalf of an incompetent adult. However, you may still treat such a patient if the treatment would be in their best interests. "Best interests" go wider than best medical interests, to include factors such as the wishes and beliefs of the patient when competent, their current wishes, their general well-being and their spiritual and religious welfare. People close to the patient may be able to give you information on some of these factors. Where the patient has never been competent, relatives, carers and friends may be best placed to advise on the patient's needs and preferences.

12. If an incompetent patient has clearly indicated in the

past, while competent, that they would refuse treatment in certain circumstances (an 'advance refusal'), and those circumstances arise, you must abide by that refusal.

Address for correspondence
Department of Health
PO Box 77
London
SE1 6XH
UK

Chapter 2
Depression

Guidelines for Depression

Reference   Guidelines for depression *Health & Ageing* (Suppl 1) (2000)

Purpose

Report of a consensus group meeting held in London, October 1999. The journal *Health & Ageing* has developed a series of guidelines of relevance to older people. The document summarizes the views of a small invited group of health professionals, and is intended to raise awareness and promote good practice.

Summary

The main emphasis of the guidance is aimed at primary care. Points made are as follows:

- Depression is not a normal concomitant of the ageing process
- The presentation may be overlooked or complicated by comorbid anxiety or dementia
- There may be problems with treatment because of age-related pharmacokinetic changes leading to increased adverse effects, or there may be interactions with other medications
- Prevalence and diagnosis of depression is discussed, along with use of suitable rating scales
- Goals of treatment include providing early and effective treatment to reduce risk and relieve symptoms, treating associated physical conditions, restoring normal function and reducing social isolation.
- Effective treatments include antidepressants and cognitive behaviour therapy
- Newer antidepressants are preferred; GPs recommended to become familiar with up to four antidepressants
- The importance of adequate dosage of drugs is discussed, also strategies for patients who fail to respond to treatment. These include increasing the dose of antidepressant, switching to a different class of drug, specialist referral, and the addition of lithium, though ECT is not mentioned.
- Measures to predict and possibly prevent suicide are important
- Prevention of depression is important – consider primary, secondary and tertiary aspects of prevention
- Finally, costs of care are elevated because of health service usage, impact upon families and need for benefits and other services.

In conclusion, depressive illness is eminently treatable. It is beholden on all those who come into contact with the elderly to recognize those at risk of depression. The cost of antidepressant medication is only a small part of the overall cost of health care for depression, and there are sizeable non-healthcare costs also to be taken into account. It is important that narrow cost perspectives are not adopted and that wider issues like social care, carer involvement, and the costs of treatment failure and non-concordance need to be considered. Appropriate management of depressive illness will prevent its excess morbidity and mortality, improve quality of life and reduce healthcare costs.

Address for correspondence

Health & Ageing
Medicom (UK) Ltd
Churston House
Portsmouth Road
Esher
Surrey KT10 9AD
UK

Diagnosis and Treatment of Depression in Late Life

Reference   Lebowitz BD, Pearson JL, Schneider LS, Reynolds CF 3rd, Alexopoulos GS, Bruce ML, Conwell Y, Katz IR, Meyers BS, Morrison MF, Mossey J, Niederehe G, Parmelee P (1997) Diagnosis and treatment of depression in late life. Consensus statement update. *Journal of the American Medical Association* 278: 1186–90

Purpose

This paper represents an update on the consensus guidelines published in 1992 on the treatment of depression in late life.

Summary

Five main points were considered.

How does depression in late life differ from depression earlier in life? What are the sources of heterogeneity in late-life depression? How prevalent is depression in the elderly, and what are its risk factors?

These questions were discussed under onset and course of depression, comorbidity and disability, subsyndromal depressions in the elderly, and sex and hormonal issues. It is recognized that depression can start early and extend into old age, or can start *de nouveau* later in life. Late-onset depression is more likely to have a chronic course and is associated with a variety of brain abnormalities such as white matter changes and ventricular enlargement with associated cognitive impairment. It was noted that depression starting later in life with cognitive impairment, even when that cognitive impairment is reversed with antidepressants, is a predictive factor for the development of dementia. The comorbidity between depression and vascular disease was emphasized. The clinical profile of patients with vascular disease is often characterized by motor retardation, lack of insight and impairment of executive functions.

It is documented that depression and associated physical illness increases the levels of functional disability and reduces the prospects for successful rehabilitation. Repeated studies have underscored the fact that treatment for depression is safe, even in the presence of comorbid physical illness. A number of immune function abnormalities have been observed in people with late-life depression.

It is emphasized that a clinically significant depression in older people is a spectrum, with rates of up to 27% being described for sub-syndromal depressions. (A variety of synonyms have been suggested, such as subclinical depression, mild depression, minor depressive disorder or sub-dysthymic depression.) These sub-syndromal disorders are associated with an increased risk of major depression, physical disability, high use of health services and medical illness. The importance of health care professionals identifying and treating these syndromes is noted.

It is noted that one of the most striking findings in psychiatric epidemiology is that women have higher rates of depression than men, with it being suggested that estrogen cannot only be helpful in the treatment of depression but may also be a protective factor against its expression.

What constitutes safe and effective treatment for late-life depression? What are the indications and contraindications for specific treatments?

These are discussed under the categories efficacy, adverse effects, psychotherapy and long-term treatment. There are comparatively few trials examining the trials of antidepressants in older people. SSRIs seems to be as effective as tricyclics, but there is a suggestion that the SSRI placebo difference may not be that great, and one study suggests that the tricyclic nortriptyline may in fact be better than fluoxetine in patients with medical illness. Elderly people tolerate SSRIs better than tricyclics. There is no evidence that older people are more sensitive than their younger counterparts to the side effects of medication, but it is noted that SSRIs are metabolized in the liver and there is a real chance of drug interaction in older people. Drop-out rates for patients in clinical trials of SSRIs are about a third to a half of those of patients treated with tricyclic drugs. Generally, the effectiveness of SSRIs over tricyclics is probably greater because of the ease of use of the drugs – less dosage adjustments, different adverse events, profiles of greater acceptance. In relation to psychotherapy, psychotherapeutic approaches have been successful in treating older patients with depression. With regard to long-term treatment, evidence supports the treatment of elderly people for at least 6 months; those with first episode illness for 12 months; and for those with recurrent episodes, generally long term treatment should be of the same type and intensity as that which was successful in the acute phase, often in contrast to prevailing practice.

What are the patterns of health service use for late-life depression? What are the obstacles to the provision of adequate treatment?

It has been well documented that major depression leads to excess use of medical services and greater health care costs.

What are the benefits of recognizing and adequately treating depression in late life? What are the consequences of unrecognized or inadequately treated depression in late life?

The association between completed suicide and major depressive illness is well recognized in older people, and the increase in suicide in the elderly is now well documented. The importance of physicians asking about suicidal thoughts in older patients who present with symptoms of depression is underscored.

What are the most promising questions for future research?

The most important issue here includes the understanding of the causes and correlates of treatment non-response or partial response, with the expectation that treatment algorithms will be developed. The importance of psychotherapeutic treatments in older people who are physically ill was emphasized, and the benefits of early intervention need to be fully assessed.

Conclusions

The main conclusion is that significant progress in the understanding of the nature of clinical course and treatment of late-life depression has been achieved since the earlier consensus. The association of late onset depression with brain abnormalities and mutual reinforcement of depression and functional disability, and the clinical importance of sub-syndromal depression, is emphasized.

Address for correspondence

Barry D Lebowitz PhD
National Institute of Mental Health
5600 Fishers Lane
Rock 18-101
Rockville, MD 20857
USA

blebowit@nih.gov

Recognition and Management of Depression in Late Life in General Practice

Reference   Katona C, Freeling P *et al* (1995) Recognition and management of depression in late life in general practice: consensus statement. *Primary Care Psychiatry* 1: 107–13

Purpose

To provide advice on the recognition and management of depression in late life, published partly to coincide with the UK Royal College of Psychiatrists' 'Defeat Depression' Campaign.

Summary

The guidelines considered a number of questions regarding depression in late life:

- Does late-life depression differ from depression in early adult life?
- How common is depression in late life?
- Which older people are at particular risk of depression?
- How best can depression be screened for in old age?
- Why and how often is depression missed in older people?

Other points considered included:

- Suicide and depression in late life, a summary of management strategies, both drug and non-drug
- How long treatment should continue
- Seeking specialist help and outcomes.

The main findings emphasize that diagnosis is difficult in older people since thoughts of death, fatigue, loss of libido, sleep disturbance and pains may all occur frequently, even in the absence of depressive symptoms.

Generalized anxiety symptoms usually respond to treatment of depression, but anxiety symptoms should be regarded as depression until proven otherwise. The prevalence of depression is around 15% in people aged over 65. Attenders in general practice have prevalence rates of about twice this, and unexplained frequent attendance may itself indicate a likelihood of depression.

Loss events such as bereavement, retirement, loss of health and reduction of mobility may precipitate depression, particularly in vulnerable individuals.

The Geriatric Depression Scale is recommended by the Royal College of Practitioners for use within the over-75 health check.

Although GPs are usually aware of the depressive symptoms of their elderly patients' experience, this is not usually reflected either in case note recording of symptoms of diagnosis, or in the initiation of treatment.

Frequent review is necessary and although a threshold for specialist psychiatric referral with avoidance of uncritical prescription of hypnotics and analgesics is recommended, most antidepressants are relatively safe in overdose.

Some older people are subject to side-effects of tricyclic antidepressants, particularly urinary retention, confusion and postural hypotension and falls.

Cognitive behavioural and brief dynamic therapies are effective in depression in late life; age should not be a factor in deciding these treatments.

Hospital evidence suggests that continuing antidepressants substantially reduces relapse rates for at least 2 years.

Referral to a specialist should be for diagnosis and/or management, with the intention that the specialist accepts responsibility for a patient's care.

Patients with severe agitation, a high suicide risk and life stupor require urgent specialist management.

As many as 31% of people remain depressed at 3-year follow-up. Failure to recover is associated with both shortened life expectancy and reduced quality of life. Continuing treatment will improve prognosis.

The primary care team is in a position to detect depression, provide a range of physical and psychosocial treatments, and carry out the indefinite monitoring that is required after the patient has recovered.

Conclusions

Depression in late life is evidently treatable and it is important that health services should be able to identify and manage this common disorder. The role of primary care teams is crucial in this respect, since they are in a position to detect depression, provide a range of physical and psychosocial treatments, and carry out the indefinite monitoring that is required after the patient has recovered. However, to do this effectively they need the advice and support of specialist mental health services, and a well-organized infrastructure of social care provision. Further education of both primary care teams and the general public to improve awareness of depression and its treatment is also needed.

Address for correspondence

Professor Cornelius Katona
Department of Psychiatry
UCL Medical School
Wolfson Building
Middlesex Hospital
London W1A 8AA, UK

Clinical Practice Guidelines on Depression

Reference   The American Medical Directors Association (1996)

Purpose

The aim of the guideline is to improve the quality of care delivered to patients in long-term care facilities, and to guide physicians, other practitioners and staff in assessing and managing depression in patients residing in long-term care settings. This guideline is based on the Agency for Health Care Policy and Research guidelines (*Depression in Primary Care – Detection and Diagnosis*, volume 1, (Clinical Practice Guideline No. 5) and *Depression and Primary Care – Treatment*, Volume 2, (Clinical Practice Guideline No. 5)). The recommendations are adapted to focus on application in the long-term care and institutional settings.

Summary

The guideline provides recommendations with respect to recognition, diagnosis and treatment of depression:

1. *Recognition.* Each patient should be assessed for a history of depression and examined for current signs and symptoms of depression. If the patient has no signs or symptoms of depression, then he/she should be evaluated for risk factors. If the patient has risk factors, these should be documented in the medical records. If no risk factors are found, the patient should be monitored periodically for the development of risk factors and for signs or symptoms of depression.
2. *Diagnosis.* If a diagnosis of depression is made, it should be decided whether a workup would be medically helpful and appropriate. A workup would evaluate possible medical causes of depression or medications that might produce the signs and symptoms of depression. Other conditions mimicking depression should also be considered. If signs and symptoms of depression are present and/or the Geriatric Depression Scale, Cornell Scale for Depression in Dementia, or the CES-D is positive, then DSM-IV criteria should be applied to strengthen the diagnosis of a major depression.
3. *Treatment.* When treating a patient with depression, the multidisciplinary team should generate a care plan. Medication and psychotherapy should be considered. The drug choice depends on the coexisting medical condition, side-effect profile, prior response, age and costs. Sedating anticholinergic drugs should be avoided. ECT may be considered if delusions are prominent, if the patient's condition is rapidly deteriorating, or if antidepressant treatment is not tolerated or has failed.

Address for correspondence

American Medical Directors Association
10480 Little Patuxent Pkwy, Suite 760
Columbia, MD 21044
USA

www.amda.com/

Detection of Depression in the Cognitively Intact Older Adult

Reference   University of Iowa Gerontological Nursing Interventions Research Center, Research Dissemination Core (1998)

Purpose

To improve detection of depression in medically compromised cognitively intact older adults in nursing homes. The potential benefits for detecting depression in the cognitively intact elderly are that it may improve quality of life and decrease the length of hospitalization.

Summary

The guideline recommends that within 72 hours of admission, each patient should be assessed for cognitive impairment using the Mini Mental State Examination. If the patient scores 23 or above, a short form of the Geriatric Depression Scale (S-GDS) should be administered. If the patient scores below 23 on the MMSE it should be established whether this is an acute change in mental status or the typical mental status for this individual. The Cornell Scale for Depression in Dementia and the Apparent Emotions Rating scale can be used to assess depression in cognitively impaired older adults.

It is recommended that the cut-off score on the S-GDS be increased to 8 to minimize false positives in the medical setting. If the patient scores 8 or greater on the S-GDS, a physician and/or geriatrician/psychiatrist should be contacted to assess the patient formally.

If the patient scores below 8 on the S-GDS, the patient's mood, sleep and appetite should be monitored. If symptoms continue, the MMSE and SGDS should be repeated every other day. Patients who score below (i.e. are subsyndromal) are at high risk for developing major depression and must be watched closely.

Address for correspondence

Copies available from:
The University of Iowa Gerontological Nursing Interventions Research Center
Research Dissemination Core
4118 Westlawn
Iowa City, IA 52242-1009
USA

www.nursing.uiowa.edu/gnirc

Chapter 3
Other disorders

APA Practice Guidelines for the Treatment of Patients with Delirium

Reference   American Psychiatric Association (1999)

Purpose

The purpose of the guideline is to assist the psychiatrist in caring for patients with delirium and to summarize information regarding the care of the patient with delirium. The practice guideline was developed under the auspices of the Steering Committee on Practice Guidelines. Key features of this process included a comprehensive literature review and the development of evidence tables, initial drafting by a working group which included psychiatrists with research and clinical expertise in delirium, the production of multiple drafts with widespread review, final approval by the APA assembly and board of trustees, and a planned revision at 3–5 year intervals. These guidelines are not specifically developed for elderly people but are for all individuals who develop delirium, regardless of age.

Summary

The recommendations in the practice guidelines fall into three categories for endorsement:

- Category 1 – recommendation with substantial clinical confidence
- Category 2 – recommendation with moderate clinical confidence
- Category 3 – recommendation which is made on the basis of individual circumstances.

The practice guideline defines delirium as primarily disturbance of consciousness, attention, cognition and perception, but it can also affect sleep, psychomotor activity and emotions. The guideline makes recommendations in three areas; psychiatric management, environmental and supportive interventions, and somatic interventions.

Psychiatric management. Psychiatric management is an essential feature of treatment, and should be implemented for all patients with delirium. Psychiatric management includes: coordinating care of the patient with other clinicians; identifying the underlying cause; initiating immediate interventions for urgent general medical conditions; providing treatment to address the underlying etiology of the delirium; assessing and ensuring the safety of the patient and others; assessing the patient's psychiatric status and monitoring it on an ongoing basis; assessing individual and family psychological and social characteristics; establishing and maintaining a supportive therapeutic stance with the patient, family and other clinicians; educating the patient's family and other clinicians regarding the illness; providing post-delirium management to support the family and patient; and providing education regarding risk factors for future episodes.

Environmental and supportive interventions. These interventions are generally recommended for all patients with delirium, and are designed to reduce or eliminate environmental factors that exacerbate delirium. They include providing an optimal level of environmental stimulation, reducing sensory impairments, making environments more familiar, and providing environmental cues that facilitate orientation.

Somatic interventions. The choice of somatic interventions for delirium will depend on the specific features of a patient's condition, the underlying etiology of the delirium and associated comorbid conditions. Antipsychotic medications are often the pharmacological treatment of choice. Haloperidol is more frequently used because it has few anticholinergic side effects, few active metabolites and a small likelihood of causing sedation and hypotension. Benzodiazepine treatment is generally used for delirium caused by alcohol withdrawal or sedative hypnotics.

Address for correspondence

American Psychiatric Association
1400 K Street NW
Washington DC 20005
USA

Acute Confusion/Delirium

Reference University of Iowa College of Nursing, Gerontological Nursing Interventions Research Center, Research Dissemination Core (1998)

Purpose

To provide guidelines for assessment and management of acute confusion/delirium in elderly patients. The guidelines are intended for both clinicians and nurses. The guidelines were developed on the basis of a consensus of experts.

Summary

The guidelines recommend that proper assessment of the patient for acute confusion is the first step. Assessment involves both admission and ongoing surveillance, with identification of individuals at high risk of acute confusion. Factors associated with increased risk of acute confusion include the following: emergency admission or admission from an institution; older age; underlying cognitive impairment; ADL impairment; polypharmacy; abnormal body temperature; low blood pressure; symptomatic infection; sensory impairment; history of falls; pain, poor social contact, dehydration.

Admission and surveillance assessment should pick up those at high risk of acute confusion. Prompt and appropriate identification of acute confusion is the cornerstone of intervention. Once acute confusion has been identified, it is vital to recognize and treat the associated or underlying causes. Physiological support should be provided and a specific communication strategy should be employed, such as using short, simple sentences, speaking slowly and clearly, identifying oneself by name at each contact, repeating questions if necessary etc. Particular recommendations regarding the environment, sound, light, and psychosocial interactions are also made in the guideline. Regarding behavioral management interventions, it is recommended that restraints be avoided if possible. Medication should be limited as much as possible, but if it is necessary to control disruptive behavior, low-dose high-potency neuroleptics or low-dose high-potency benzodiazepines are recommended.

Address for correspondence

University of Iowa Gerontological Nursing Interventions Research Center
Research Dissemination Core
4118 Westlawn
Iowa City, IA 52242-1100
USA

www.nursing.uiowa.edu/gnirc

Schizophrenia and Older Adults

Reference   Cohen CI, Cohen GD, Blank K, Gaitz C, Katz IR, Leuchter A, Maletta G, Meyers B, Sakauye K, Shamoian C (2000) Schizophrenia and older adults. *American Journal of Geriatric Psychiatry* 8: 19–27

Purpose

To identify research and policy areas that need to be addressed regarding schizophrenia in older adults.

Summary

The USA Group for the Advancement of Psychiatry, Committee on Ageing believes that a crisis has emerged with respect to the understanding and nature of treatment of schizophrenia in older people. Six research and policy recommendations are made following an examination of the epidemiology, social functioning, physical health, and treatment and service provision for this group.

Recommendations

The number of older persons with schizophrenia will increase dramatically over the ensuing decades, and therefore policymakers must begin to reorder research and service priorities to anticipate this growth. Our overview of the status of older persons with schizophrenia reveals that in many instances there are appreciable alterations in psychopathology, neuropsychological status, social functioning and health that distinguish them from younger persons with the disorder. Nevertheless, the research literature on ageing and schizophrenia is sparse, and many key areas must be addressed if we are to meet adequately the psychiatric, medical and social needs of this group. Failure to respond to these issues may result in costly, inappropriate services that fail to satisfy the subjective or objective needs of this population. The review indicates that some of the most critical research and policy areas that must be addressed are:

1. To establish more clearly which factors determine subjective and objective mental, physical and social well-being of older persons with schizophrenia so as to provide optimal functioning in the community, and in order to determine how persons with schizophrenia compare with older persons with other psychiatric disorders and with older persons with no mental illness.
2. To clarify which factors predict levels of psychopathology, such as positive and negative symptoms, depression and neuropsychological deficits among older persons with schizophrenia, and to determine the most effective long-term treatment of these symptoms.
3. To clarify factors that would improve illness behavior and service utilization of older persons with schizophrenia, and to contrast older schizophrenic persons with older persons with other psychiatric disorders, as well as those persons without mental illness.
4. To elucidate those factors that determine burden among caregivers of older persons with schizophrenia and compare them with caregivers of persons with other disorders, to develop models that will help enhance the natural support systems of schizophrenic persons.
5. To determine what is the optimal service mix for persons with comorbid physical and chronic mental illness.
6. To establish economic models for funding care for older persons with chronic mental illness. Emphasis must be placed on the role Medicare, Medicaid and managed care will play in supporting these services and, with respect to the latter, how 'carve-in' models (combined mental/physical health care) compare with 'carve-out' models (distinct mental health and physical health care).

Methodologically, addressing these questions poses several challenges. First, with respect to sampling, it will be necessary to develop samples that capture the range of residential, clinical, geographic and sociodemographic diversity of the older schizophrenic population. Thus, samples must include community and institutionalized persons, and persons living with families as well as those living independently and in supervised settings. Many of the earlier 'classic' studies were based on long-term follow-up catamnestic evaluations of persons who had been institutionalized. However, proportionately more schizophrenic persons may not be hospitalized, and among those who have been hospitalized, follow-ups are difficult because of rapid changes in the composition of many urban areas, as well as greater family mobility; thus, stratified sampling from many geographic areas may be more practical. Moreover, it is critical to obtain well-matched control groups so as to avoid errors due to sociodemographic confounds such as social class or cultural background.

A second issue will be to develop the appropriate instruments to operationalize the variables in the questions listed above. Until recently, very few instruments had been validated for older schizophrenic persons. However, community-based and institution-based studies by the Jeste and Davidson research groups, respectively, have used an array of scales to assess psychopathology, cognition, and psychosocial functioning, which can provide the basis for future work. Depending on the questions to be asked, more extensive instruments can be introduced and tested. Hence, the scaffolding is now in place to begin to construct a knowledge base from which the needs of older persons with schizophrenia can be addressed.

Address for correspondence
Dr C Cohen
SUNY Health Sciences Center at Brooklyn
Box 1203
450 Clarkson Avenue
Brooklyn, NY 11203
USA

Late-onset Schizophrenia and Very Late Onset Schizophrenia-like Psychosis: An International Consensus

Reference   Howard R, Rabins PV, Seeman MV, Jeste DV (2000) Late-onset schizophrenia and very-late-onset schizophrenia-like psychosis: an international consensus. *American Journal of Psychiatry* 157: 172–8

Purpose

Through a systematic review of the literature and publication of a consensus statement from an international group of experts in the field, the consensus statement summarized the findings in terms of diagnosis and nomenclature of treatment guidelines in future research directions in late-onset schizophrenia.

Summary

Schizophrenia, whether of early or late onset, from childhood to old age, is fundamentally heterogeneous and presumably consists of a group of related illnesses. In order to better understand the pathophysiology and aetiology of the schizophrenias, to overcome difficulties associated with a lack of consistency in diagnostic criteria and nomenclature and to develop multicenter studies of late-onset schizophrenia, an international consensus has been articulated with respect to specific definitions and current research questions. We believe that there is sufficient evidence to justify recognition of two illness classifications: late-onset (onset after the age of 40 years) schizophrenia and a very-late-onset (onset after 60) schizophrenia-like psychosis.

The case for heterogeneity with increased onset age

Schizophrenia-like psychoses, which cannot be attributed either to an affective disorder or focal or progressive structural brain abnormality, can arise at any time in the life cycle between childhood and old age. The expression of such psychotic symptoms shows greatest variation when onset age is at both extremes of life. Since the aetiologies and the distinctive pathophysiologies of schizophrenia are at present unknown, variations in epidemiology, symptomatology, pathophysiology and treatment response with age at onset can help to provide important clues to causative risk factors.

Epidemiology

Female sex is associated with later age at onset. Incidence curves for men and women are different, and some preliminary data suggest three adult peaks that correspond to early adult life, middle age and old age. Very-late-onset cases may arise in the context of sensory impairment and social isolation.

Symptomatology

Early-and late-onset cases are more similar than different in terms of symptoms (especially positive symptoms). The only study of a large representative sample found almost no differences up to the age of 60 but in clinical samples, extreme old age at onset is associated with a low prevalence of formal thought disorder and affective blunting and a higher prevalence of visual hallucinations. Differences in symptoms profiles with onset across the age span do not necessarily imply differences in pathophysiology or aetiology; they could represent cohort differences or age-associated central nervous system differences independent of the illness. Alternatively, similar symptoms could arise from different aetiopathological processes.

Pathophysiology

There is no evidence that a progressive dementing disorder is associated with onset in middle or old age. Regardless of onset age, schizophrenia is associated with a generalized cognitive impairment relative to age-matched unaffected subjects. No difference in type of cognitive deficits has been found between early- versus late-onset cases. Later onset of schizophrenia is, however, associated with somewhat milder cognitive deficits, especially in the areas of learning and abstraction/cognitive flexibility. Brain imaging findings are essentially similar regardless of onset age. In the late-onset group, no excess of focal structural abnormalities, such as areas of MRI signal hyperintensity are more prevalent in patients with late-onset affective disorders than in age-matched comparison subjects.

Aetiology

Familial aggregation of schizophrenia is more common in earlier and middle-age onset than in very-late-onset cases. There is no satisfactory evidence that later age at onset of these disorders breeds true. Some studies suggest familial loading for affective disorders in patients with later-onset schizophrenia. The prevalence of a family history of Alzheimer's disease, vascular dementia, dementia with Lewy bodies or apolipoprotein E genotype is not higher in later-onset cases.

Age at onset cut-off points

The available data suggest that categorization by specific age at onset ranges is relatively arbitrary. Although consensus was achieved, members of the group could not reach unanimity on either the presence of age cut-offs or where they should be set. There was general agreement that cut-offs have clinical utility and act to stimulate research effort. Epidemiological evidence is strongest for a cut-off at age 60 to define the very-late-onset group. Some clinical studies support another cut-off at age 40 although epidemiological data suggest that this age point may be too high for the middle-age onset group.

Nomenclature

After much discussion, a consensus was reached that cases in which onset occurs between age 40 and 60 be called late-onset schizophrenia and that cases in which onset occurs after the age of 60 should be called very-late-onset schizophrenia-like psychosis. The purpose of this nomenclature is to clarify the position of these patients and to stimulate more research, rather than to put a closure on this issue.

Assessment and treatment

Regardless of age at onset, psychiatric and medical examinations and available investigative procedures should always be obtained to exclude identifiable aetiologies. If available, brain imaging should be obtained in cases of late-onset schizophrenia and very-late-onset schizophrenia-like psychosis. The presence of sensory impairments and social isolation should be ascertained and appropriate remedial action taken if found. The place of non-pharmacological treatments has not been adequately investigated but access to these therapies should not be prejudiced by age. Psychological management may reduce distress associated with psychotic symptoms and facilitate a therapeutic relationship, within which commencement and compliance with medication can occur.

Antipsychotic drugs are the mainstay of therapy. Drug treatment should be started at very low doses and increase in dose should be made slowly. Typical late-onset patients will respond to dose amounts that are about one-quarter to one-half those given to early-onset patients. Very-late-onset cases may respond to dose amounts as low as one-tenth of those used in young adults. Use of depot medication at very low doses may be successful in ensuring compliance. With the exception of clozapine, whose use is problematic in older patients, the atypical antipsychotic agents are clearly advantageous in the treatment of late-onset patients because of the reduced likelihood of extrapyramidal symptoms and tardive dyskinesias for which elderly patients are at higher risk.

Future directions
Epidemiology

Epidemiological studies should use standardized criteria but should have no criterion that excludes a diagnosis of schizophrenia based on late age at onset. When comparisons are made by age at onset, first-onset episodes should be clearly defined. Because cases of late-onset schizophrenia and very-late-onset schizophrenia-like psychosis are uncommon, multicentre studies are necessary.

Long-term follow-up studies can provide valuable information and test the hypothesis that patients tend to have a similar course regardless of age at onset. Both risk and protective factors should be sought.

Symptomatology

Because late-onset schizophrenia has a higher proportion of women than early-onset illness and gender interacts with symptom variables such as emotional expressiveness and social activity, it is important to control for gender when comparing the prevalence of symptoms by age at onset. Comparison of symptoms of idiopathic cases of schizophrenia with symptoms of cases secondary to known causes at a range of onset ages would be fruitful.

Pathophysiology

Specific cognitive models should be tested in patients with onset in childhood, young adulthood, middle age and old age to establish whether identified cognitive abnormalities are truly similar across the age-at-onset span. Cognitive tests, which are increasingly sophisticated and allow for fine distinctions of performance, should be used in combination with functional brain imaging in order to test hypotheses of differential neurocircuitry involvement. In very-late-onset cases, the possible role of sensory impairment should be further explored.

Aetiology

Brain imaging studies that involve adequate numbers of subjects and that use SPECT, PET and functional MRI should be conducted with patients across the age-at-onset span. Diffusion tensor imaging has promise as a technique to examine white matter structure. Testing models of disconnection and misconnection across a wide range of onset ages should be considered. The role of oestrogen withdrawal should be further explored, as should genetic, viral, birth injury and degeneration-related factors. Large existing data sets should be explored with reference to late- and very-late-onset groups.

Treatment

Appropriately designed clinical trials of pharmacological and psychological treatments are required. SPECT and PET receptor occupancy studies that compare early- and late-onset cases would be valuable for understanding drug action and treatment response. Multisite studies of combined pharmacological and psychosocial/behavioural management approaches – with meaningful outcome measures such as quality of life and activities of daily living functioning – are warranted.

Address for correspondence
Dr R Howard
Section of Old Age Psychiatry
Institute of Psychiatry
De Crespigny Park
Denmark Hill, London SE5 8AF, UK

Guidelines for the Management of Parkinson's Disease

Reference   Bhatia K, Brooks DJ, Burn DJ, Clarke CE, Playfer J, Sawle GV, Schapira AHV, Stewart D, William AC (1998) Guidelines for the management of Parkinson's disease. *Hospital Medicine* 59: 469–80

Purpose

The guidelines present the first UK-specific advice for the management of Parkinson's disease, including a treatment decision tree.

Summary

Key points are summarized under the categories of the diagnosis of Parkinson's disease, the role of drug treatment of Parkinson's disease, recommendations for surgical treatment of Parkinson's disease, and the role of the multidisciplinary team.

Diagnosis of Parkinson's disease

- Parkinson's disease is a clinical rather than a pathological diagnosis.
- There is often some uncertainty in the diagnosis of Parkinson's disease, particularly in its early stages.
- The use of acute L-dopa and apomorphine challenge tests is not recommended, as their sensitivity is lowest in *de novo* patients.
- It is advantageous for *de novo* patients to be referred to specialist centres for diagnosis and management.
- Early bulbar or gait problems should alert the physician that atypical disease may be present.
- Neurological conditions with clinical features similar to Parkinson's disease include multiple system atrophy, progressive supranuclear palsy, post-encephalatic parkinsonism, essential tremor, multiple infarct state and drug-induced parkinsonism.
- Imaging techniques have greatly enhanced the understanding of the disease, but no technique provides 100% specificity for Parkinson's disease.

The role of drug treatment of Parkinson's disease

- The rationale for current drug use in Parkinson's disease is the correction of abnormal neurotransmitter function, primarily in dopaminergic neurons, with resulting symptomatic relief.
- L-dopa in combination with a peripheral decarboxylase inhibitor is the most effective symptomatic treatment available for Parkinson's disease, but its long-term use is associated with disabling complications even if *de novo* patients are treated with controlled-release preparations.
- Because of the complications associated with L-dopa therapy, it is prudent to delay treatment with L-dopa provided that adequate relief can be achieved with other treatment strategies.
- Treatment with dopamine agonists, amantadine, selegiline and anticholinergics can help to delay introduction of L-dopa. Dopamine agonists are recommended as a first-line alternative to L-dopa in appropriate patients.
- Nigrostriatal degeneration leads to increased dopamine turnover and potential production of neurotoxic free radicals. To date no drug has been shown to have clinical efficacy as a neuroprotective agent, but potential neuroprotective agents are being investigated.

Recommendations for surgical treatment of Parkinson's disease

- There are three targets for neurosurgery in the brains of Parkinson's disease patients; the thalamus, the globus pallidus and the subthalamic nucleus (STN).
- Unilateral thalamotomy may be considered for patients with severe (functionally disabling) drug-resistant unilateral tremor. Bilateral thalamatomy is not recommended.
- Pallidotomy relieves dyskinesias and allows the use of a higher L-dopa dose in responsive patients.
- Subthalamotomy is experimental at present.
- Thalamic stimulation is at least as effective as thalamotomy for the relief of tremor, and may be used bilaterally.
- Bilateral STN stimulation appears to be highly effective in relieving parkinsonism, but may cause involuntary movements in some patients.

The role of the multidisciplinary team

- The parkinsonian patient requires a continuum of care, which is best provided by a multidisciplinary team.
- GPs should ideally refer all patients with suspected Parkinson's disease to a movement disorder specialist before starting therapy.
- The multidisciplinary team should be led by a consultant specializing in movement disorders, who should ensure that team members are appropriately trained.
- The multidisciplinary team must include professionals with specialist expertise (including a Parkinson's disease specialist nurse) and the person(s) caring for the patient.

- The specialist nurse, based in a dedicated clinic, provides an essential link between the patient and members of the multidisciplinary team.
- The multidisciplinary team and GPs should agree local guidelines and working practices.

Address for correspondence

Professor D Brooks
Consultant Neurologist
Imperial School of Medicine
Hammersmith Hospital
London W12 0NN
UK

Standards of Medical Care for Older People: Expectations and Recommendations

Reference   **British Geriatrics Society (1997)**

Purpose

This guidance confirms areas of care which are good, and sets benchmarks of service for the establishment and maintenance of appropriate services. The document outlines both standards that should be available at all times, and expectations that are reasonable and achievable.

Summary

Standards cover several areas, including:

- general information and communication
- achieving the best possible health
- illness
- recovery and rehabilitation
- discharge from hospital (see BGS/ADSS/RCN guidance)
- special health services for older people
- community and social services
- changing home
- support during terminal illness
- drugs and medicines
- transport to and moving around hospital and GP surgeries
- the older person's responsibilities.

Health services should aim to:

1. Promote good health and wellbeing and to prevent and lessen illness, disability and long-term infirmity among older people
2. Treat illness when it does happen
3. Enable older people to lead as full and independent a life as possible as active members of the community
4. Provide a comprehensive health and social service to support people in their own homes
5. Ensure appropriate provision of institutional care when it is required
6. Ensure that dignity is preserved and distress minimized at all times
7. Ensure that service effectiveness and efficiency are promoted through clinical audit, research and development
8. Ensure that training and high professional standards are established and maintained by all staff.

The standards have been endorsed by various other organizations, including Age Concern, the Association of Directors of Social Services, the College of Occupational Therapists, Royal College of General Practitioners, Royal College of Nursing, Royal College of Physicians (London), Royal College of Physicians and Surgeons of Glasgow, Royal College of Physicians (Edinburgh), Royal College of Psychiatrists, and the Royal College of Speech and Language Therapists.

Address for correspondence

The British Geriatrics Society
1 St Andrew's Place
Regent's Park
London NW1 4LB
UK

Chapter 4
General statements

National Service Framework for Older People

Reference   http://www.doh.gove.uk/nsf/olderpeople.htm March 2001, Department of Health.

The National Service Framework for Older People is a comprehensive strategy to ensure fair, high quality, integrated health and social care services for older people. It sets out a programme of action and reform to address the problems often faced by older people such as discrimination against them, failing to treat them with dignity and respect and thereby allowing organisational structures to become a barrier to poor assessment of need and access to care. The overarching aim is to improve the services delivered to older people.

Summary

The contents of the National Service Framework for Older People is in 5 chapters.

Chapter 1   Introduction
Chapter 2   Eight standards
Chapter 3   Local Delivery
Chapter 4   Ensuring progress
Chapter 5   National Support to underpin local action.

Some 369 references are contained in the NSF. The eight standards are summarised in the table.

The aim of Standard 7 (Mental Health in Older People) is to promote good mental health in older people and to treat and support those older people with dementia and depression. The chapter is divided into a number of headings including the rationale for the importance of the subject, a note of the key interventions needed i.e. promoting mental health, early recognition and management of mental health problems and access to specialist care. There are descriptions of the important aspects of depression and dementia, care pathways for dementia, depression and confusional state and a service model for a specialist mental health service.

Three actions are suggested: the National Health Service and local authority councils should review the local system of mental health services in older people, including the arrangements for mental health promotion (Standard 8), early detection and diagnosis, assessment, care and treatment planning and access to specialist services.

The second standard is that they should review current arrangements in primary care and elsewhere for the management of depression and dementia and agree and implement local protocols across primary care and specialist services including social care. In time this should be extended to cover all mental health problems in older people.

The third standard is that current arrangements should be reviewed in primary care and elsewhere for the management of dementia in younger people and agree and implement a local protocol across primary care and specialist services including social care.

The eight National Service Framework standards are:

Standard One: Rooting out age discrimination

NHS services will be provided, regardless of age, on the basis of clinical need alone. Social Care services will not use age in their eligibility criteria or policies, to restrict access to available services.

Standard Two: Person-centred care

NHS and social care services treat older people as individuals and enable them to make choices about their own care. This is achieved through the single assessment process, integrated commissioning arrangements and integrated provision of services, including community equipment and continence services.

Standard Three: Intermediate care

Older people will have access to a new range of intermediate care services at home or in designated care settings to promote their independence by providing enhanced services from the NHS and councils to prevent unnecessary hospital admission and effective rehabilitation services to enable early discharge from hospital and to prevent premature or unnecessary admission to long-term residential care.

Standard Four: General hospital care

Older people's care in hospital is delivered through appropriate specialist care and by hospital staff who have the right set of skills to meet their needs.

Standard Five: Stroke

The NHS will take action to prevent strokes, working in partnership with other agencies where appropriate.

People who are thought to have had a stroke have access to diagnostic services, are treated appropriately by a specialist stroke service, and subsequently, with their carers, participate in a multidisciplinary programme of secondary prevention and rehabilitation.

Standard Six: Falls

The NHS, working in partnership with councils, takes action to prevent falls and reduce resultant fractures or other injuries in their populations of older people.

Older people who have fallen receive effective treatment and rehabilitation and, with their carers, receive advice on prevention through a specialised falls service.

Standard Seven: Mental health in older people

Older people who have mental health problems have access to integrated mental health services, provided by the NHS and councils to ensure effective diagnosis, treatment and support, for them and for their carers.

Standard Eight: Promoting an active healthy life in older age

The health and well-being of older people is promoted through a co-ordinated programme of action led by the NHS with support from councils.

Further copies: Dept of Health, PO Box 777, London SE1 6XH, United Kingdom

Out in the Open: Breaking Down the Barriers for Older People

Reference   Gazdar C, Pettit R (2000) UK Department of Health Public Services Productivity Panel

Purpose

To help UK Departments deliver improvements in productivity, efficiency and the quality of services.

Summary

Introduction

1. The Public Services Productivity Panel (PSPP) was established in 1998 'to help Departments deliver improvements in productivity, efficiency and the quality of services, not least the targets set out in their Public Service Agreements'.

2. The Department of Health agreed that one of the Department's projects should look at the scope for local councils to improve efficiency through better commissioning of social services for adults, particularly for older people. This was because:

   - Commissioning is critical to delivering key Government policy aims – to help people to live independently and to make sure that services fit individual needs. It is through commissioning that local councils specify and secure services. Commissioning practice may determine how many older people, for example, are enabled to live independently at home or enter long-term residential care.

   - Local councils spend over £6 billion a year on personal social services for adults, including residential care. There are significant variations between councils in the unit cost (and pattern) of commissioned services. For example, the average weekly unit cost of supporting older people in nursing care in England in 1997–98 was £286, ranging from £100 or less a week in a small number of councils to more than £450 a week in others. The weekly cost for a supported resident aged 65 or over in independent sector residential care during the same period varied from less than £100 to over £400 (the average cost being £217). The hourly cost of home help/care for individual councils in 1997–98 varied from less than £6 in some to more than £15 in others, with the average hourly unit cost being £8.80.

   - The new flexibilities in the Health Act 1999, including pooled budgets and joint commissioning, offer opportunities to develop innovative and integrated services that provide greater choice for service users and more efficient use of local government and NHS resources. To maximize these benefits, local councils need to be ready to challenge traditional approaches to commissioning.

   - In the consultation on the findings of the National Beds Inquiry (NBI), the Department of Health has invited views on the future development of intermediate care, i.e. promoting care closer to home for older people. An active policy to build up intermediate care would require a major expansion of social care (and health) services to help maintain people in their home communities, facilitate early discharge from hospital, promote active rehabilitation after an acute episode and support a return to normal community-based living, wherever possible. Effective and efficient local authority commissioning would be a vital factor in delivering this.

3. The project focused on commissioning for older people rather than other adults because:

   - There is a growing concern that older people are not best served by current arrangements and service options.

   - There are high numbers of inappropriate admissions of older people to residential and nursing homes.

   - There is a lack of well-developed diversionary and rehabilitative services aimed at this group.

   - Issues of volume and demand have tended to result in service- rather than needs-led responses.

   - There is an under-developed approach to commissioning arrangements – both at a strategic (political/senior management) and operational (care managers/social workers) level.

   - There is a lack of information around value for money of services purchased.

Aim and objectives of the project

4. The project aimed:

   - To test the effectiveness of direct intervention in replicating good practice and securing sustainable improvements in the efficiency, quality and range of local social services authority commissioning for older people.

5. The objectives of the project were to:

   - Identify the problems associated with ineffective commissioning and their causes (including both inappropriate commissioning of long-stay residential care and inefficient commissioning arrangements).

- Identify and test solutions, both by commissioning different service models and by improved commissioning arrangements.
- Measure the improved outcomes for users and efficiency gains (including cost savings for commissioners).
- Make recommendations on the usefulness of direct interventions with individual councils, compared with written guidance or other traditional means.

Project sites

6. A deliberately diverse group of four pilot sites was recruited to participate in the project. Differences included size, geography, environmental factors, diversity of population served, political composition and historically varied approaches to implementation of community care. However, the sites' willingness to participate in a collaborative and experimental way was critical.

Barriers to good commissioning

7. Those identified in the pilot sites were:
   - An inflexible organizational culture

- Poor or inadequate management information
- Lack of monitoring frameworks
- Lack of or unwillingness to undertake joint or multi-agency commissioning
- Poor standards of assessment at the individual level
- Underdeveloped alternatives to residential care
- Resistance to encouragement of independent sector providers
- Difficulty in recruiting sufficient numbers of home care staff
- Poor involvement of users, carers and front-line staff in the commissioning process.

Work undertaken during the project

8. This included external facilitation by the Nuffield Institute for Health; the establishment of multidisciplinary focus groups and workshops: advice and guidance to the pilot councils from the Department of Health's Social Care Policy Branch and Social Care Regions; and one-off meetings between the Chair of the project's steering group and elected members of the councils and senior local NHS staff.

9. Examples of the initiatives undertaken by the pilot sites are:

Service	Date opened	Outcome
Social re-enablement unit	24 Jan 2000	6 people discharged – 4 home, 2 with minimal domiciliary care packages
Rehabilitation and recuperation project	Project manager appointed. Due to open spring/ summer 2000	Anticipated: 11% diversion from residential care – savings to be calculated
Delegation of placement decisions (with set targets)	Commenced Sept 1999	Targets met: 6–10% reduction in admissions to residential care
Retrospective care audit of 50 placements	November 1999	Has demonstrated diversion possibilities if alternatives had been available
Specialized nursing home rehabilitation services	Tender process completed and providers selected	Anticipated: reduction in long-term care dependency by 25%–50%. Estimated saving, for example, of £5200 p.a. for each person diverted from nursing to residential care
(1) Intake and assessment team + (2) Multidisciplinary assessment	(1) Pilot in planning stages (2) 3 pilots up and running	Expected diversion from residential care of up to 30%
Extra care facility	Currently undergoing best value review. Looking to open 2001/2002	Diversion from residential care
Rapid response team	29 Nov 1999	Estimated savings of £43,200 in first 3 months

Conclusion

10. The four diverse project sites all benefited from direct intervention visits and were able to make rapid changes that have made a difference to the lives of some older people. The recent nature of the service developments means that only now are data becoming available. The sites can increasingly provide more data – including financial savings achieved and projected. Whilst the project is very much a work in progress, there are emerging findings.

Emerging findings

11. The most significant are:
   - External intervention can be a powerful stimulus for local change.
   - Greater direct involvement from the centre, e.g. the Department's Social Care Policy Branch, can raise the profile and perceived importance of commissioning.
   - Face-to-face contact with commissioners can be more helpful than traditional forms of guidance, such as Departmental circulars.
   - Guidance customized for local use, e.g. when transcribed on to floppy disks, can be more effective than traditional forms.
   - It is important to involve independent sector providers at the outset of the commissioning process.
   - Guiding commissioners through the plethora of available good practice and research can bring positive results.
   - Raising the profile of the Department's Social Care Regions and making local councils more aware of the support on offer can bring about improved commissioning.

12. The project has provided a better understanding of how certain indicators suggest policy and practice issues that would respond to direct intervention. The intention is to continue with the project for the next 3 months. This will:
   - Provide information to confirm or adjust the emerging findings
   - Guide dissemination and future roll-out of the project's approach and results.

Address for correspondence

Roger Pettit
Department of Health
211 Wellington House
133–155 Waterloo Road
London SE1 8UG
UK

www.doh.gov.uk/outintheopen

The Way to go Home: Rehabilitation and Remedial Services for Older People

Reference   Audit Commission (2000) The way to go home: rehabilitation and remedial services for older people. Audit Commission Publications

Purpose

To highlight the role of rehabilitation for older people.

Summary

Older people are major users of health and social services:

- Two-thirds of hospital beds are occupied by people aged 65 or over
- Two-thirds of social services expenditure on people over 75 goes on residential and nursing home care
- The numbers of older people are growing, increasing pressures on these services.

Effective rehabilitation can help people to stay at home or return home after hospital, and reduce admissions to residential and nursing homes. It requires a range of services . . .

- Multidisciplinary teams working in people's own homes to prevent admissions and help people home after hospital
- After acute care, further specialist medical and nursing attention as part of an intensive multidisciplinary programme
- Once medical problems have stabilized, places in homely settings for more active rehabilitation and confidence building

. . . and well-integrated care

- Processes and services should be clearly linked
- Care should be co-ordinated by a multidisciplinary team within the framework of a multi-agency joint investment plan.

In practice, services are variable . . .

- In areas visited, the number of rehabilitation beds per person over 75 varied by a factor of five
- Therapy time per bed varied from a few minutes to nearly an hour per day.

. . . and there are major gaps:

- Only one-third of areas have multidisciplinary teams to support people at home, reducing hospital emergency admissions, re-admissions and length of stay
- Only one-half of trusts have a stroke unit, despite strong evidence of their effectiveness
- Just one-half of areas have places away from hospitals for active rehabilitation, costing half as much as hospital places.

The rehabilitation programme needs co-ordinating . . .

- Comprehensive assessment is essential, but under one-quarter of areas use joint health and social services documentation
- Over one-quarter of stroke patients reported poor communication
- Out of 15 areas, two used combined notes and only one a single care plan.

. . . and therapists need to be used effectively:

- Good information is required to help managers deploy therapists to where they are most needed
- Workforce planning is needed to provide more staff
- Assistants and helpers can release professionals to work more effectively.

Agencies need to plan together, sharing a 'whole-systems' approach and making use of new financial flexibilities. Effective rehabilitation services promote the well-being of older people and help to reduce waiting lists and winter pressures.

Address for correspondence

Audit Commission Publications
Bookpoint Ltd
39 Milton Park
Abingdon OX14 4TD
UK

The Coming of Age: Improving Care Services for Older People. National Report

Reference   Audit Commission (1997) Audit Commission Publications

Purpose

The Audit Commission oversees the audit of local authorities and the National Health Service Agencies in England and Wales. This report consists of an amalgamation of two related studies: continuing care (a review of the arrangements for people leaving hospital who require ongoing or continuing care), and the commissioning of community care (a review of how local authorities commission services for those who are assessed as needing care).

Summary

Mapping needs and services

1. Health authorities and social services departments must map needs and the services available to meet them. They should share this information with each other as the basis for joint planning and commissioning.
2. Health authorities and trusts should review whether older people are currently being admitted to hospital beds because alternative services are not available and identify what alternative services are needed.
3. Social services should review their spending patterns, use of residential and nursing homes, use of home care and any limits to placements, and make adjustments in this mix where needed.

Strengthening management information

4. Health and social services authorities should support their mapping processes by introducing information systems that allow them to update their maps on a regular basis.

Working with service providers

5. Health authorities should work with trusts to develop new forms of provision to reduce admissions to hospital by providing care in alternative ways, and explore ways of improving rehabilitation after treatment where appropriate.
6. Social services should actively seek better relationships with independent sector providers through a better understanding of the provider's point of view.
7. Social services should develop their contracting and funding mechanisms to improve the balance between security for providers and more favourable terms for themselves. In particular, they should explore ways of rewarding providers for quality and innovation.

Assuring quality

8. Social services should develop more watertight monitoring arrangements to ensure effective and high quality service delivery, co-ordinating the resources that they have and adding to them where necessary.

Address for correspondence

Audit Commission
1 Vincent Square
London SW1P 2PN
UK

The Discharge of Elderly Persons from Hospital for Community Care: A Joint Policy Statement

Reference   British Geriatrics Society, Association of Directors of Social Services & Royal College of Nursing (1995)

Purpose

This statement is issued in the spirit of informing those committed to commissioning and providing the best quality of health care for older people. Whilst set in the legal context of required local frameworks, it seeks to identify and promote the specific values and standards of policy, care practice and discharge planning required to ensure a quality service to elderly people.

Summary

The document sets out the underlying rationale for the policy statement, and lists key principles and values underlying its recommendations. The recommendations are in two sections – the hospital experience and discharge.

The hospital experience

1. Discharge planning should commence, whenever possible, from the point at which a patient is admitted.
2. The patient should be treated and cared for in an atmosphere which recognizes their abilities, encourages re-enablement and promotes the confidence to maximize their capacity for self-care.
3. The family and other informal carers are an integral part of the treatment, rehabilitation and care programme.
4. Whilst it is recognized that the majority of elderly people in hospital are treated by departments other than those specifically specializing in the medicine of old age, the principles, values and practices espoused in this joint statement should inform the care they receive wherever the treatment is based, especially general medical wards, acute trauma ward, urology wards, general surgery wards and accident and emergency departments.
5. The specialists in the medicine and nursing of old age have a key role within hospitals to inform not only the standards of care and treatment of older people but also discharge decisions. Routine involvement by consultant geriatricians and multidisciplinary teams in all hospital departments with a high proportion of elderly people is desirable, but clearly has resource implications.
6. Specialists in the medicine of old age within multidisciplinary professional teams have the key role in determining and, wherever possible, ensuring that the community care assessment is not undertaken when the client is in an unstable clinical or psychological state and that the maximum level of function is achieved before life-long decisions are taken.
7. There is, nevertheless, a corporate responsibility to ensure that there is the least possible delay in hospital discharge consistent with informed patient choice.

Discharge

1. Discharge should only follow a multidisciplinary assessment.
2. The components determining a quality discharge process are set out in the form of a checklist (appended to the document).
3. The date for the determination of an agreed post-discharge care plan and when it will be reviewed needs to be established in all cases before discharge, including determining whether the specialist in the medicine of old age has a continuing role in the treatment and care planning process.
4. Where return to the patient's previous home situation is agreed not to be feasible as a consequence of a multidisciplinary assessment in which the patient has been engaged, then a very sheltered housing, residential or nursing home placement should be considered.
5. The least intrusive and most independent supporting situation should be sought. A new living situation should be arranged from the individual's own home or whilst they are resident in hospital, whichever is more suitable for the individual older person and their significant others.
6. For patients with complex conditions or multiple problems, the discharge process may be prolonged due to slow recovery. Transitional arrangements may be required, but these should not preclude the future provision of a complex package of care.
7. Where the multidisciplinary health care team have assessed an older person to have a need for continuous nursing, then they should not be subsequently reassessed/redesignated without the involvement of the specialist nurse with expertise in the health care of older people.

Addresses for correspondence

Dr Alistair Main
Chair, Policy Committee
BGS
Queen Elizabeth Medical Centre
Edgbaston
Birmingham B15 2TH
UK

Martin Shreeve
Chair, ADSS Services for Elderly People Committee
Social Services Dept
Civic Centre
Wolverhampton WV1 1RT
UK

Pauline Ford
Nursing Advisor for Older People
RCN
20 Cavendish Square
London W1M 0AB
UK

Organization of Care in Psychiatry of the Elderly: A Technical Consensus Statement

Reference   World Health Organization, World Psychiatric Association (1997)

Purpose

This is a technical consensus statement on the organization of care in psychiatry of the elderly, jointly produced by the Geriatric Psychiatry Section of the World Psychiatric Association and WHO and several other collaborators. The objectives of the document are to:

- promote debate at the local level on the mental health needs of older people and their caregivers
- describe the basic components of care for older people with mental disorders and their coordination
- stimulate, assist and review the development of policies, programmes and services in psychiatry of the elderly according to the framework of the WHO Primary Health Care Strategy
- encourage the continuous evaluation of all policies, programmes and services to older people with mental disorders.

The statement is divided into five parts:

1. *General principles:* these make some general statements. For example, all people have the right of access to a range of services which can respond to their health and social needs, and the needs should be met appropriately for the cultural setting and in accordance with scientific knowledge and ethical requirements. Services should be designed for the promotion of mental health in old age as well as for the assessment, diagnosis and management of mental disorders. Governments should work with non-governmental agencies, and have a responsibility to improve and maintain the general mental health of older people and to support their families and carers.

2. *Specific principles:* these are described as needing to be comprehensive, accessible, responsive, individualized, transdisciplinary, accountable and systemic (CARITAS).

3. *Care need section:* includes headings on prevention, early identification; comprehensive medical and social assessment (including diagnosis), continuing care, support and review of the individual and carers, information advice and counselling; regular breaks (respite) advocacy, residential care and spiritual and leisure needs.

4. *Descriptors of components of services:* includes sections on community mental health teams for older people, inpatient services, day hospitals, outpatient services, hospital respite care, continuing hospital care, liaison services, primary care, community and social support services, and prevention.

5. *Conclusions:* this concludes that the document is not meant to be either totally comprehensive or prescriptive, and that detailed descriptions of methods of treatment and care have not been included. The statement identifies care needs of older people with mental disorders and suggests some of the ways by which these are currently met in some parts of the world. Where this is not the case, it is argued that people responsible for health care policy development and implementation should take note of the requirements cited and act accordingly, that components of the services should be integrated and coordinated, and that the attainment of best possible quality of life of elderly people with mental disorders is the ultimate guiding principle and organization of care. It also emphasizes that good services should always be underpinned by good research, evaluation and training.

Psychiatry of the Elderly: A Consensus Statement

Reference   Jointly produced by WHO and the Geriatric Psychiatry Section of the World Psychiatric Association (1996) World Health Organization

Purpose

The objectives of the statement are not only to define geriatric psychiatry, but also to encourage the development of this discipline for the benefit of the elderly.

Introduction

The population of old (and particularly very old) people is increasing rapidly throughout the developed and developing world. This reflects improving health and social conditions, and is a cause for celebration. Most older people remain in good mental as well as physical health, and continue to contribute to their families and to society.

This notwithstanding, some mental illnesses (such as the dementias) are particularly common in old age; others differ in clinical features and/or present particular problems in management. Social difficulties, multiple physical problems and sensory deficits are also common. Appropriate detection and management require specialist knowledge and skills as well as multidisciplinary collaboration.

Priority needs to be given to these mental illnesses which can cause a great deal of stress not only to older people themselves, but also to their families. This is aggravated by changing family structures. There is also an increasing number of older people living alone. Appropriate interventions for the major mental illnesses of old age can often either treat them effectively or at least substantially improve the quality of life of patients and their families.

The rise in numbers of older people with mental health problems has necessitated the development of the specialty of psychiatry of the elderly. The emergence of the specialty of psychiatry of the elderly has helped to raise the status of this vulnerable group, and has also fostered research which offers hope for better treatment and outlook and provides the opportunity for training students in all health and social care related disciplines.

This summary of the scope of psychiatry of the elderly is intended to promote awareness of mental health problems in older people, to initiate or improve the provision of services, and to encourage teaching and research in the area.

Definition and assessment

Psychiatry of the elderly is a branch of psychiatry, and forms part of the multidisciplinary delivery of mental health care to older people. The specialty is sometimes referred to as geriatric psychiatry, old age psychiatry or psychogeriatrics.

Its area of concern is the psychiatry of people of 'retirement' age and beyond. Many services have an age cut-off at 65, but countries and local practices may vary; several specialist services include provision for younger people with dementia. The specialty is characterized by its community orientation and multidisciplinary approach to assessment, diagnosis and treatment.

An elderly patient suffering from mental health problems often has a combination of psychological, physical and social needs. This implies that individual assessment management and follow-up requires collaboration between health, social and voluntary organizations and family carers. Mental health problems in old age are common, and an understanding of the principles involved in their identification and management should be an integral part of the general training of all health and social care workers.

Progress in the field must be evidence-based and founded on rigorous empirical research with which practitioners should aim to keep up-to-date.

Past experience and behaviour may influence whether a person develops mental illness and how such illness presents itself. Multiple losses (death of relatives/friends, declining health, loss of status, etc.) in old age may be particularly important, though many older people remain resilient despite multiple adversity.

The specialty deals with the full range of mental illnesses and their consequences, particularly mood and anxiety disorders, the dementias, and the psychoses of old age and substance abuse. In addition, the specialty has to deal with older people who developed chronic mental illness at a younger age. At any rate, psychiatric morbidity in old age frequently coexists with physical illness, and is likely to be complicated by social problems. Older people may also have more than one psychiatric diagnosis.

The above factors, together with the biological, social and cultural changes associated with ageing, may significantly alter the clinical presentation of mental illness in old age. Current diagnostic systems (ICD-10, DSM-IV etc) do not fully allow for these factors.

The diagnostic approach is essentially similar to that used in other age groups. There are nevertheless some differences. Older people are often frightened by unfamiliar diagnostic investigations. They should have their initial assessment in their home or other familiar setting wherever possible. It is particularly important to obtain a collateral history. Invasive or stressful tests should only be undertaken where their results might alter management or to fulfil family needs for diagnostic answers.

Many mental illnesses in old age can be treated successfully. Some (particularly the dementias) are chronic and/or progressive. Appropriate intervention can nonetheless contribute to improving quality of life. A diagnostic formulation should emphasize abilities as well as deficits and incorporate the meaning given to the illness by the patient and the family. Both assessment and intervention may involve overlap between professional roles as well as coordination between services.

Treatment

The objectives of treatment may include restoration of health; improving quality of life, minimizing disability, preserving autonomy and addressing supporters' needs are equally valid. Treatment must be adapted to the individual patient's needs and to available resources. Its delivery usually requires cooperation between the multidisciplinary professionals involved, as well as involvement of informal supporters. Early detection and intervention may improve prognosis, and education is required to counteract the therapeutic pessimism of both professionals and patients.

Treatment must pay due regard to individual patient's wishes; dignity and autonomy must be respected. Consent to treatment by patients no longer competent to make such decisions raises important ethical and legal issues.

Older people with mental illnesses (particularly depression) may take longer to respond to treatment than their younger counterparts. Functional psychiatric illnesses in late life have a high rate of relapse; close follow-up and continued treatment may reduce this.

Older people are particularly vulnerable to the side effects of psychotropic drugs. Consideration must also be given to age-related changes in drug handling. Interactions between psychotropic drugs and older patients' comorbid physical illnesses (and their treatment) are also common. Coexistent physical problems in older people with mental illness must be treated; this may facilitate treatment of the mental illness.

Treatments to improve cognitive functioning in people with dementia and/or modify the course of the disease are being actively researched. Vascular dementia may be prevented or slowed by treatments that reduce risk of stroke.

All psychotherapeutic techniques (e.g. supportive, psychodynamic and cognitive/behavioural) may be used with older people. Adaptations may be necessary to take into account any sensory or cognitive deficits.

Therapeutic interventions to encourage autonomy include retraining in daily living skills and improving safety at home. Provision of practical support and information including social and legal rights' advice to patients and their

supporters make an important contribution.

Organization of services

Most older people with mental health problems are cared for by their families and/or friends with support from the primary care team, which also provides continuity of care. The primary care team (as well as other service providers) needs to be able to refer to the old age psychiatry service when further opinions and advice are needed and/or for direct specialist care.

The multidisciplinary specialist service in old age psychiatry can include a range of professionals such as doctors, nurses, psychologists, occupational therapists, physiotherapists, social workers and secretarial staff, who should meet regularly to coordinate and discuss new referrals and current caseload. The team should have an identified leader.

Initial assessments should wherever possible be in the patient's home; family members and the primary care team should be involved. The assessment should result in the formulation of a care plan and follow-up arrangements with clear objectives, defined responsibilities for multidisciplinary team members and the primary care team (usually with a single designated 'key worker'). This should include the provision of support, information and advice to carers.

In order for the specialist service to work effectively, a range of resources needs to be available and accessible. These include an acute inpatient unit, rehabilitation, day care, respite facilities and a range of residential care for people no longer able to live in their own homes. Reciprocal availability of advice between psychiatry of the elderly and general medical and (where available) geriatric medicine is important. Links with community facilities are important (e.g. day centres and support groups for carers as well as for patients themselves).

A comprehensive service in psychiatry of the elderly should be patient-centred and achieve sufficient coordination between its elements to ensure continuity of care. The service should be integrated into the health and social welfare system, and is dependent upon an adequate social, political, legal and economic framework.

Quality assurance must be a priority within all parts of the service. This is particularly important to ensure respect for the needs and wishes of those older people who are unable to express them fully.

Training

The specialty of psychiatry of the elderly requires a grounding in general psychiatry and in general medicine as well as training in the specific aspects of both psychiatric and medical conditions as they occur in older people. Psychiatry of the elderly should be taught in the variety of settings in which it is practised.

Training schemes for all health and social care workers

should include a component on mental health care of older people. Training in mental health care of older people should be offered at both undergraduate and postgraduate level and also during continuing professional development. Education and information about mental health care of older people should be offered to the general public and to carer groups. The development of appropriate training manuals with culturally appropriate material should be achieved for all groups of professionals and carers.

Research
Research in old age psychiatry covers a wide range, including molecular biology, epidemiology, neurochemistry, psychopharmacology, health service research (including evaluation of innovative community projects) and ethics.

Research in this area provides a unique opportunity for cross-fertilization between disciplines, is crucial for the advance of the specialty, and may have benefits beyond its domain. Workers in the field need training in research methods, as well as time and opportunity to pursue research.

The Quality Challenge. Caring for People with Dementia in Residential Institutions in Europe: A Transnational Study

Reference   The quality challenge. Caring for people with dementia in residential institutions in Europe (1999) Alzheimer Scotland

Purpose

The study explores comparisons of the European countries' quality of residential institutional care for people with dementia. It aims to provide baseline information on the role of institutional care in the continuum of care of people with dementia, to evaluate the effectiveness of different policy approaches, to promote awareness of effective policy innovations, and to promote the diffusion and adoption of innovative approaches throughout the European Union. Institutional care was defined as *accommodation for five or more people who need care, where care is provided 24 hours a day by paid staff, with the intention of long-term care for an extended period.*

Conclusions and recommendations

In spite of advances in recent years, institutional care for people with dementia remains an under-developed area of policy. Good quality care was generally seen to be non-standardized and tailored to the needs of the individual with dementia, whose choices should be respected. Although there were examples of good practice in key components of individualized care, there was a need for further development and implementation. Small-scale models of institutional care were considered appropriate for people with dementia. Examples of good practice included 'supported housing', with an emphasis on 'ordinary housing', and care provided separately. One approach in traditional institutions is to create small units within the larger institution, which has some of the advantages of both large- and small-scale models. This is an area where it is important for countries to share experiences and to disseminate models which have proved effective. The next stage of this project will contribute to the dissemination of models of policy and practice.

Policy makers in individual countries are best placed to formulate specific policies and practices geared to their own systems and the most salient issues in their countries. However, the project recommends that, in developing such measures, the following issues are specifically addressed:

- Better integration of health and social services in a comprehensive approach to the spectrum of care for people with dementia, of which institutional care forms a part
- Planning for future needs for culturally appropriate institutional care for people from minority ethnic communities and with diverse lifestyles
- Development of quality assurance systems alongside monitoring of minimum standards, especially in Italy and Spain
- Effective implementation of multidisciplinary assessment and individual care planning, including consultation with the main informal carer
- Recognition of the value of the continuing contribution of informal carers, and of the relationship of people with dementia with local community groups such as their church or club, to the quality of their life
- Development of measures to protect and promote rights of people with dementia
- Empowerment of people with dementia and/or their representatives
- Development of methods to understand the preferences of people with dementia and to communicate about these preferences in verbal and non-verbal ways
- Programmes for training, particularly specialized dementia care training
- Specific policy measures and resources to support family and community involvement and promote social integration of people with dementia in institutional care
- Small-scale local units to promote such community integration
- Design of the built environment with features that aid orientation and understanding
- Promotion of privacy and dignity of people with dementia through provision of single bedrooms with en suite facilities and adequate private space.

In the near future, the need for residential institutional care for people with dementia will increase significantly. Good quality care will most appropriately be provided in small-scale living units, of which there is a growing diversity of models to be adapted to particular circumstances. The importance of seeing the person with dementia as an individual whose choices should be respected must be central to all policy developments. Ensuring good quality services is essential for people with dementia, who are not always able to complain or exercise their rights.

Address for correspondence

Alzheimer Scotland
Action on Dementia
22 Drumsheugh Gardens
Edinburgh EH3 7RN
UK

Forget-Me-Not: Mental Health Services for Older People. National Report.

Reference   Audit Commission (2000) Forget-me-not: mental health services for older people. Audit Commission Publications

Purpose

The UK audit commission oversees the external audit of local authorities and the National Health Service in England and Wales. As part of this function, the commission is required to undertake studies to enable them to make recommendations to improve the economy, efficiency and effectiveness of services provided by these bodies. This is the first in a series of reports with a common theme of promoting independence for older people.

Summary

The key recommendations to improve the help given to older people with mental health problems are as follows.

In the early stages:

1. GPs and other primary care staff should provide information, support and competent advice.
2. Information about the services available locally, presented in a way that can be understood easily by local people, should be distributed to GP surgeries and other public places.
3. Local mental health professionals should provide training and support for GPs and primary care teams, making particular efforts to contact those who refer very few people.

Once specialist help becomes necessary, a range of services is needed, including:

4. Assessment by members of a community mental health team (CMHT), where possible, at home on at least one occasion.
5. Provision that is balanced in favour of home-based services.
6. A range of specialist community-based staff – ideally with specialist home-care workers. Service managers should consider training home-care staff who express an interest in developing skills in this area.
7. Day provision for time-limited assessment and treatment (day hospitals) as well as long-term care (day centres), with an appropriate mix of staff to meet needs, and planned jointly by health and social care agencies.
8. Respite care in a range of settings, including at home, with some places reserved for emergency situations.

Those who can no longer cope at home need:

9. Hospital admission for people with psychiatric and behavioural problems that cannot be managed in any other setting, with close links to physical health care services – with admissions limited by effective community services.
10. Residential and nursing homes, supported by mental health specialists, to enable them to care for highly dependent individuals, and with a strong emphasis on quality.
11. NHS-funded continuing care for those in greatest need, as determined jointly by health and social services agencies.

Such complexity needs to be managed through:

12. Good co-ordination between health and social care, with integrated teams of professionals who have ready access to a range of flexible services.
13. Effective care planning for individuals, through the Care Programme Approach or a similar method.
14. Effective information sharing between practitioners, preferably with shared files.

All of the elements of a comprehensive service need to be drawn together at a strategic level with:

15. Clear goals, including the intended balance between home-based, day, outpatient and hospital services.
16. Good quality information to inform planning, including monitoring of service quality.
17. An approach that promotes innovation and works towards jointly commissioned services by health and local authorities, as emphasized by national policy.

Address for correspondence

The Audit Commission
1 St Vincent's Square
London SW1P 2PN
UK

www.audit-commission.gov.uk

Standards for Mental Health Services for Older People

Reference   Finch J, Orrell M (1999) Health Advisory Service

Purpose

This is one of several sets of standards developed by the Health Advisory Service 2000 to underpin its work of conducting systematic external reviews of services. Each set of standards was derived by using a consistent methodology, involving an extensive literature review and input from a multidisciplinary advisory network. It is intended that this first edition of standards will be modified in the light of its application in practice and future service and policy developments.

Summary

The document consists of a list of standards, each underpinned by a list of criteria relevant to the standard, with references wherever there is supporting published evidence. The standards are grouped into four levels, which mirror the organizational structures within which services operate. Figure in brackets indicate the number of standards under each heading.

Level I: Service delivery

1. Individual needs assessment   (3)
2. Individual care planning   (7)
3. Clinical interventions   (1)

Level II: Organization of care

1. Access   (1)
2. Range of services   (4)
3. Day care/community treatment facilities   (4)
4. Inpatient care   (6)
5. Long-term care   (3)
6. Respite care   (1)
7. Health and social care interventions   (2)
8. Information for users, carers and others   (2)

Level III: Intra-agency organizational issues

1. Policies   (6)
2. Overall management of services   (1)
3. Staffing levels and skill mix   (2)
4. Staff support and supervision   (2)
5. Staff morale   (1)
6. Staff training and education   (2)
7. Clinical governance, quality assurance and audit   (5)
8. Information management   (1)

Level IV: Planning, integration and commissioning

1. Needs assessment   (1)
2. Strategies   (2)
3. Implementation, monitoring and quality assurance   (4)
4. Resource allocation   (1)
5. Service agreements   (3)
6. Joint planning   (4)
7. Joint working   (3)
8. Commissioners' and service planners' expertise and
   knowledge   (1)
9. Research   (2)

Addresses for correspondence

Health Advisory Service
46–48 Grosvenor Gardens
London SW1W 0EB
UK

Pavilion Publishing (Brighton) Ltd
8 St George's Place
Brighton
East Sussex BN1 4GB
UK

Consensus Statement on the Upcoming Crisis in Geriatric Mental Health

Reference   Jeste V, Alexopoulos A, Bartels SJ, Cummings JL, Gallo JJ, Gottlieb GL, Halpain MC, Palmer BW, Patterson TL, Reynolds CF, Lebowitz BD (1999) Consensus statement on the upcoming crisis in geriatric mental health. *Archives of General Psychiatry* 56: 848–53

Purpose

The statement reflects the outcome of a workshop held in March 1998 to discuss the current state of affairs in the upcoming crisis in geriatric mental health and to recommend the research agenda.

Summary

In the USA, the number of people over the age of 65 with psychiatric disorders will rise from 4 million in 1970 to 15 million in 2030. The current health care system serves mentally ill older people poorly, and is unprepared for the upcoming crisis in geriatric mental health. Studies of prevention and translation of findings from bench to bedside, large-scale intervention trials with meaningful outcome measures and health service research are suggested, with new methods of clinical research training involving specialists and primary care clinicians and the lay public. The document is divided into several sections.

1. The current state of affairs
   - epidemiology of mental illness in older adults
   - present system of mental health care delivery for older adults.
2. Suggested research agenda
   - prevention
   - translational research
   - intervention studies
   - Health Services research
   - training.

Conclusions

To recommend a multi-pronged approach beginning with the formulation of 15–25 year plan for research into mental disorders in elderly people. The key points in the research agenda include: reduction of risk factors for cerebrovascular disease; trial of the prevention of Alzheimer's disease; the development of a biological marker to give a definitive diagnosis of Alzheimer's disease with appropriate modifications of diagnostic criteria to incorporate specific aspects of mental health in older people; studies of pharmacological and non-pharmacological approaches to mental health disorders including psychotherapies and cognitive therapies. Studies to assess the impact of managed care of older people with mental health problems should be undertaken, and training should be directed at closing the gap between clinical practice and the research literature.

Address for correspondence

Dr Dilip Jeste
University of California
San Diego
VA San Diego Health Village Dr
San Diego, CA 92161
USA

djeste@ucsd.edu

No Secrets: Guidance on Developing and Implementing Multi-Agency Policies and Procedures to Protect Vulnerable Adults from Abuse

Reference   Department of Health (2000)

Purpose

This is the product of a multi-agency steering group led by the UK Department of Health, along with the Home Office, the Association of Chief Police Officers, the Association of Directors of Social Services, the voluntary sector and academic bodies. The aim of *No Secrets* is to ensure that key local agencies, particularly but not solely health, social services and the police, are able to work together to protect vulnerable adults from abuse, by developing local multi-agency policies and procedures. The coordinating role falls to social services departments, who are expected to ensure that local multi-agency codes of practice are developed and implemented by the end of October 2001.

Summary

This applies not only to older people, but to all vulnerable persons aged 18 or over. Abuse includes: physical abuse, sexual abuse, psychological abuse, financial or material abuse, neglect and acts of omission, and discriminatory abuse.

Sections of the report include:

1. Defining who is at risk and why
   - which adults are 'vulnerable'?
   - what actions or omissions constitute abuse?
   - who may be the abuser(s)?
   - in what circumstances may abuse occur?
   - patterns of abuse
   - what degree of abuse justifies intervention?
2. Setting up an inter-agency framework
   - identify all the responsible and relevant agencies
   - establish multi-agency management committee
   - clarify roles and responsibilities within and between agencies
   - develop procedures and formulate guidance
   - implement equal opportunity policies and antidiscriminatory training
   - balance the requirements of confidentiality with need for information sharing
   - identify mechanisms for monitoring and review.
3. Developing inter-agency policy
   - sets out items that should be included in policies
   - lists the guiding principles that agencies should adhere to.
4. Main elements of strategy
   - list of items to be included in strategy
   - training for staff and volunteers
   - commissioning of services and contract monitoring
   - confidentiality and information sharing.
5. Procedures for responding in individual cases
   - objectives of an investigation
   - content of procedures
   - management and coordination of response to allegation of abuse, including procedures for receiving a referral; investigation; record keeping; assessment; person against whom allegation is made; staff discipline and criminal proceedings; decision making.
6. Getting the message across
   - dissemination of information
   - rigorous recruitment practices (NB references; volunteers)
   - internal guidelines for all staff
   - information for users, carers and the general public.

Address for correspondence

Paul Mascia
Department of Health
221 Wellington House
133–155 Waterloo Road
London SE1 8UG
UK

http://www.doh.gov.uk/coinh.htm

Not Because They Are Old: An Independent Inquiry into the Care of Older People on Acute Wards in General Hospitals

Reference   (1999) Health Advisory Service

Purpose

In response to a campaign in the Observer newspaper in autumn 1997, the UK Department of Health established an inquiry, carried out by HAS 2000, into the care of older people on acute wards. The study was conducted in 16 randomly selected acute hospital wards, including direct observations of the ward environment, the quality of the patient's day, and the quality of the interactions between ward staff and older patients.

Summary

The following key themes were listed and followed by appropriate recommendations:

1. Satisfaction with care: generally lower among older people and their relatives compared with other mixed age samples.
2. Delays in admission: significant numbers admitted through A&E departments experienced unacceptably long delays.
3. Deficiencies in the physical environment.
4. Shortages of equipment and supplies, and staff time wasted in obtaining them.
5. Staff shortages.
6. Supply and quality of food and drink.
7. Feeding and nutrition: relatives frequently reported a lack of help from staff in relation to feeding.
8. Privacy and dignity.
9. Communication and pressures on staff from heavy workloads.
10. The role of the ward manager: crucial to delivery of good quality care.
11. Agreeing the boundaries of care, between staff, patients and relatives.
12. Staff attitudes towards older people: staff generally had positive attitudes about their jobs, despite feeling over-stretched and under pressure.
13. Staff–patient interactions: negative interactions can be mediated by other pressures, e.g. poor physical environment, workload, staff and equipment shortages.
14. Staff appraisal and development: personal development systems are essential to eliminate poor care.
15. Education and training: specific deficits identified in many skills, especially feeding, assessment of swallowing, management of continence problems.
16. Discharge from hospital: often problems with discharge planning and accessibility of community support.
17. Integration versus specialism: conflicting evidence, but multidisciplinary approach on specialist elderly care wards may have benefits.

Address for correspondence

Health Advisory Service
46–48 Grosvenor Gardens
London SW1W 0EB
UK

What a Difference a Nurse Makes. An RCN Report on the Benefits of Expert Nursing to the Clinical Outcomes in the Continuing Care of Older People

Reference   UK Royal College of Nursing (1997)

Purpose

A response from the nursing profession to the debate on the provision of continuing care for older people. Nurses are concerned that what they regard as health care needs are increasingly being redefined as needs for social care. This poses a threat to the quality of care provided to older people, as they may be denied access to the skilled nursing care that they in fact require. This document aims to provide means of demonstrating the value of nursing care through the measurement of outcomes from clinical practice, particularly in continuing care settings.

Summary

The general emphasis is upon a holistic approach to nursing care, which encompasses quality and life satisfaction, rather than using longevity or other disease-specific outcome measures. An alternative approach to outcome definition is presented, which centres on identifying indicators of nursing practice using case examples. A framework for analysing such case examples is offered. The approach also identifies specific nursing intervention outcomes and suggests that, to relate these to the overall quality of care, existing quality measures are used. Available and appropriate audit tools are recommended.

Measurement of outcomes requires the identification of patient outcome criteria specific to nursing. Three domains of outcome have been developed:

1. Maintenance of health status
   - maximizing health status
   - assessment of health status
   - prevention of disease complications
   - managing risk
   - rehabilitation
   - identification and relief of symptoms.
2. Prevention and relief of distress
   - essential care and palliation
   - identifying problems and coming to terms with life
   - prevention of pain
   - treatment of pain
   - mental health assessment.
3. Maximizing life potential
   - health promotion and education
   - life-long development
   - meaningful relationships
   - contribution to life

- reciprocity
- coping with adversity.

A model is suggested for identifying one's own outcome indicators:

Stage 1   How do I identify a practice example? – i.e. an incident where your intervention really made a difference to a patient's care

Stage 2   How do I reflect on the practice example? – includes describing, clarifying and learning from the experience

Stage 3   Analysing the experience and applying the matrix – matrix includes four elements; empirical knowledge, tacit knowledge, skills, experience

Stage 4   Identifying the outcome and the indicator for nursing – what were the final outcomes, and what was the indicator for nursing?

The document then goes on to discuss the particular contribution of expert nursing for older people, which offers their value in the following ways:

- understanding the influences on care, e.g. ageism, class, gender, ethnic background
- maintaining a positive, person-centred approach
- building and maintaining relationships
- skilled assessment
- intervention
- developing expert specialist nursing roles.

Finally, a selective review of available tools for measuring quality is presented. The measures outlined include the Royal College of Physicians/British Geriatrics Society CARE scheme, Monitor and Senior Monitor, Nursing Home Monitor I and II, the Quality Patient Care Scale (QUALPACS), and the King's Fund Organizational Audit for Nursing Homes (KFOA).

Additional references

Royal College of Nursing (1993) *Older People and Continuing Care: The Skill and Value of the Nurse.* RCN

Royal College of Nursing (1995) *Nursing and Older People: Report of the RCN Taskforce on Nursing and Older People.* RCN

Address for correspondence

Royal College of Nursing
20 Cavendish Square
London SW1M 0AB, UK

The Person, The Community and Dementia: Developing a Value Framework

Reference   Cox S, Anderson I, Dick S, Elgar J (1998) Dementia Services Development Centre

Purpose

Project funded by the Help the Aged and carried out by the DSDC at Stirling. This publication aims to share understanding of current knowledge and expert opinion (expert includes people with dementia, their families and caring networks), and explores how this can be made accessible to a wide range of users, carers, commissioners, providers, planners and practitioners across all sectors. The main focus is on how values inform the process of understanding dementia and negotiating the provision of care and support.

Summary

This reviews the literature on values and principles as applied to dementia and its care, also on understanding people with dementia. The methodology of the project is described, and then the framework itself, which is a graphical presentation consisting of the following five frames:

1. Frame I *A value framework for dementia.*
   This has five core values, with the person with dementia at its centre
   - maximizing personal control
   - enabling choice
   - respecting dignity
   - preserving continuity
   - promoting equity.
2. Frame II *The impact of dementia.*
   Each person with dementia has characteristics and needs
   - shared with some or all other human beings
   - arising from individual personality, history and circumstances
   - relating to the ever-changing impact of their illness.

   Dementia, whether diagnosed or not and at whatever stage, changes how people are able to manage their lives, how they see themselves and how others treat them.
3. Frame III *Personhood and communication are maintained.*
   As it progresses dementia leads to growing dependence on the emotional and practical responses of known individuals, of service providers and the community. Responding appropriately to the individual, fluctuating and progressive needs of people with dementia is a highly complex undertaking.
4. Frame IV *Empowering, negotiating and balancing.*
   The interests of family and other informal carers, like those of other individuals and organizations involved, may conflict with the interests of the person with dementia and with each other. Many factors contribute to conflict, and balancing conflicting interests requires constant negotiation and re-negotiation. Good practice and shared values can minimize the negative effects of conflict, and contribute positively to defining standards and outcomes which aim to keep the person with dementia at the centre and empower them.
5. Frame V *Ideas sheet.*
   The framework is designed for practical use with individuals in the development of person-centred care plans, as well as to provide a structure for organizational thinking on a wider canvas.

Address for correspondence

Sylvia Cox
Planning Consultant
Dementia Services Development Centre
University of Stirling
Stirling FK9 4LA
UK

Home Alone. Living with Dementia

Reference   Alzheimer's Disease Society (1994)

Purpose

Many people with dementia live alone and may be at particular risk of neglect, accident, injury or exploitation. Demographic and social changes are likely to increase numbers in this group. Report includes information from two surveys; one of consultants in old age psychiatry looking at service needs, and one of the readers of *SHE* magazine, looking at current attitudes of contemporary women in middle life.

Summary

1. There are an estimated 154 000 people with dementia in the UK living alone in the community.
2. This number is estimated to grow to 245 000 by 2011.
3. Accidents are a common cause of referral to specialist services. There is also increased risk of self-neglect, injury and exploitation.
4. Thirty-seven per cent of consultants in old age psychiatry considered the level of support for people with dementia living alone to be poor, and 63% considered it no better than adequate.
5. All people with dementia living alone will need continuing care eventually. The health service has cut continuing care beds by 40% between 1989 and 1994.
6. Most working women surveyed in *SHE* magazine look to government-funded health and social care services to be the major providers of care and financial security for elderly people.
7. Eighty-two per cent of women surveyed in *SHE* said they had not made plans for their parents in old age.

Recommendations

1. Department of Health to ensure that all local health authorities collect adequate data on people with dementia living in the community.
2. NHS Executive to establish purchasing guidelines for dementia services.
3. Community care services to be oriented towards flexible domiciliary care, with properly paid and trained workers, recognizing that those who live alone do so for 7 days a week, 24 hours a day.
4. Particular attention to the safety of people living alone.
5. Need of people living alone for long-term nursing care should be recognized.
6. Department of Health to encourage more vigilant application of health care checks for people aged 75 and over by GPs, including the Patient's Charter right to yearly home visits.
7. Department of Health to emphasize the need for early diagnosis and assessment of people with dementia by primary health care teams.

Further reference

Alzheimer's Disease Society (1994) *Safe as Houses: A Resource Booklet to Aid Risk Management.*

Address for correspondence

Alzheimer's Society
Gordon House
10 Greencoat Place
London SW1P 1PH, UK

www.alzheimers.org.uk

Dementia Care: Challenges for an Ageing Europe

Reference   European Institute of Women's Health (1999)

Purpose

The purpose of the document was to highlight the challenges posed by Alzheimer's disease and other dementias to other European member states, and emphasize the cross-country comparison of policies and practices implicit in the variation that currently exists regarding treatment of dementia and support of carers across Europe. It is emphasized that women may bear the brunt of dementia as patients and as carers in the future.

Summary

Recommendations were made under four headings.

Policy

1. Develop financial, legal and social service models for dementia to ease the burden on patients, their families and carers.
2. Encourage the collection of comparable data at a European level on the social and economic costs of dementia as a basis for policy planning.
3. Strengthen and develop voluntary services and public sector partnership models.
4. Develop legal safeguards to protect the individual rights of people with dementia.
5. Encourage the exchange of information on models of best practice between EU member states.
6. Develop policies that delay or prevent institutional care by offering a range of care and housing options, thus enabling dementia patients to remain at home or in the community as long as possible.
7. Encourage a multidisciplinary approach to dementia integrating medical, social and governmental sectors in dementia care.
8. Establish a range of care and housing options in the community that will delay or prevent institutional care.
9. Give dementia services a specific priority in the broader context of health care.
10. Develop a set of standards for the provision of home care.
11. Initiate further reports on the scientific information needs of home carers.
12. Establish specialty of 'one-stop shops' to defragmentize care, simplify procedures for carers, and provide a central contact for interfacing with relevant agencies.

If Member States are to plan for adequate services in a humanitarian and cost-effective manner, it is essential to determine the cost of dementia to the State at progressive stages of the illness for the family, the community and the health care system.

Research

1. Conduct gender-comparable studies to investigate the impact of dementia among men and women.
2. Initiate further research into psychosocial aspects of dementia and its impact on families, carers, patients and society as a whole.
3. Encourage pharmacological research for the development of useful therapies with minimal side effects.
4. Examine preventive strategies in relation to lifestyle issues, in particular, cardiovascular disease and dementia.

Education

1. Educate both public and policy-makers about dementia and emphasize the magnitude of care required, stressing that dementia is an illness amenable to care and treatment, not an inevitable process of ageing.
2. Initiate broad-based campaigns to educate clinical and social service providers and ensure the inclusion of dementia topics as a standard part of medical curricula and training, thereby ensuring timely diagnosis and treatment.
3. Educate families about early diagnosis and treatments available, while allowing them every opportunity to make decisions and arrangements for continuing care.
4. Initiate public health education regarding the benefit of lifestyle changes in reducing vascular dementia.

Quality of life and independence

The death of a dementia sufferer creates particular problems of bereavement, given the close relationship during the caring period and the lack of communication in the final stages of the disease.

1. Emphasize 'personhood' of the dementia patient, and keep treatment and care focused on preserving the quality of life for patients and maintaining their dignity.
2. Provide regular respite care and emergency support for home carers, who are themselves subject to stress-related

physical and mental illnesses.

3. Develop training programmes for voluntary and paid carers to enhance the level of care. Training courses should cover areas such as making the home safe for dementia patients, managing incontinence, feeding and bathing, time and stress management, recognizing non-dementia illness, dealing with aggression, and maintaining patient independence.

4. Provide counselling services to help carers cope with depression and the stress of care.

Care must be tailored to the needs of individuals and their families rather than to the established practices of institutions or the public system. The issue is not simply managing dementia patients, but helping them to make the most of their remaining years.

Address for correspondence

European Institute of Women's Health
9 Herbert Place
Dublin 2
Ireland

info@eurohealth.ie

www.eurohealth.ie

Right from the Start: Primary Health Care and Dementia

Reference   Alzheimer's Disease Society (1995)

Purpose

This report investigates the perception that general practitioners have difficulty with their role in helping patients with dementia and their carers to obtain access to care and services. Data are presented from two surveys, one of 2000 carers, looking at their experiences of primary cares services, and the other of nearly 700 GPs, investigating their views on the diagnosis and management of dementia.

Summary

GPs have a key role in helping people with dementia and their carers to obtain access to care. Many GPs face an increasing volume of work and inadequate local services, and they have a lack of training in dementia, so find this role difficult.

The carers' survey found:

1. When consulted by patients with a memory problem, most GPs did not give a memory test and 42% did not offer a diagnosis.
2. Of those subsequently found to have dementia, 13% were first thought by GPs to have depression and 17% 'old age'.
3. Thirty-six per cent of patients diagnosed with dementia were not referred to a specialist.
4. Sixty-nine per cent of carers found their GP helpful and supportive, but only 24% thought his or her knowledge of dementia was very good.
5. Nearly 50% of carers thought they were not given enough information about the disease. The ADS was found to be the most informative source by 45% of carers, and GPs by only 19%.
6. Nearly 60% of carers reported health problems as a result of caring, but only 32% received regular follow up from their GP.
7. Although almost half the carers were over 70 years, only 28% had been offered an annual health check.

The GPs survey found:

1. Seventy-one per cent felt they had not had adequate training in the management of dementia.
2. Over half were dissatisfied with community services and 42% thought admissions to residential care were more difficult since the 1993 Community Care Act.
3. Almost all had heard of the ADS, but only 33% were aware of their local branch.
4. Only 14% referred carers to the ADS.

Recommendations

1. Department of Health to give priority to GP training and education in the needs of people with dementia and their carers.
2. GPs to pay greater attention to the value of early diagnosis of dementia.
3. GPs to improve links with other professionals/better multidisciplinary working.
4. GPs to ensure that continuing health and social care needs of people with dementia and their carers are met.
5. Government to consider incentives for GPs to carry out over-75 health checks more thoroughly.
6. GPs and voluntary organizations to forge partnerships locally to support people with dementia and their carers.
7. The ADS to work at national and local levels to increase GP awareness of the Society and its services.

Address for correspondence

Alzheimer's Society
Gordon House
10 Greencoat Place
London SW1P 1PH
UK

www.alzheimers.org.uk

Purchasing Clinical Psychology Services: Services for Older People, Their Families and Other Carers

Reference   British Psychological Society Division of Clinical Psychology (1995) *Briefing Paper No. 5*

Purpose

This document looks at the psychological needs of older people and the psychological aspects of the health care and social care services they may receive. It sets out the aims in providing health gains through a high quality and cost-effective service. Quality standards and measures of quality are itemized. There are recommendations for the organization and staffing of clinical psychology services, and implications for the training of clinical psychologists.

Summary

Main sections deal with: (a) requirements in health and community care of older people; (b) service specifications; and (c) monitoring services.

1. Requirements include:
    *   estimating the extent of psychological need
    *   health service objectives for older people
    *   health gains and cost-effective activities
    *   enhancing health care, emphasizing care management, user and carer orientated services, working partnerships with carers, training and support for staff, and evaluating quality of care.
2. Services specifications include:
    *   core services (direct clinical work, indirect clinical work, psychological consultancy, and research and development)
    *   innovative practices
    *   organization of clinical psychology services (across various settings, including people's own homes)
    *   service standards
    *   staffing levels – for a population of 250 000, the BPS recommend two whole-time equivalents for people with dementia, plus two in support of geriatric medicine, plus others offering other services
    *   training issues.
3. Monitoring services include:
    *   outcome measures (suggested indices are listed in document)
    *   quality outcomes and service audit.

Address for correspondence

British Psychological Society
St Andrews House
48 Princess Road East
Leicester LE1 7DR
UK

Caring about Carers: A National Strategy for Carers

Reference   UK Department of Health (1999)

Purpose

Sets out the British Government's package of policy measures to support carers. In Britain, one person in eight (about 6 million people altogether) act as carers. Support to carers is seen as an effective means of helping those older people who are looked after by informal carers. The strategy applies largely, but not solely, to those providing care for older people.

Summary

The strategy has three main elements:

1. Information
   - a new charter on what people can expect from long-term care services, setting new standards
   - consideration of how to improve the consistency of charging for services
   - the carers' need for good health information
   - the NHS Direct helpline for carer information
   - Government information on the internet.
2. Support
   - carers need to be involved in planning and providing services
   - local caring organizations should be consulted
   - comment cards, advice surgeries, carers' weeks are good ways to involve carers.
3. Care
   - carers have a right to have their own health needs met
   - new powers for local authorities to provide services for carers, as well as those being cared for
   - the first focus of the new powers should be on helping carers take a break
   - a new special grant to help carers take a break
   - on top of the £750 million for prevention and rehabilitation, there will be £140 million over the next 3 years to help carers take a break, to be used in a targeted way
   - financial support for working carers to be kept under review.

The Government's carers' package also includes:

- new legislation to allow authorities to address carers' needs
- time spent caring will entitle carers to a second pension
- the Government is consulting on proposals, but by 2050 carers could receive an extra £50 per week in today's terms
- reducing council tax for disabled people being cared for
- support for neighbourhood centres, including carers' centres
- considering scope for extending help to carers to return to work
- a new census question to tackle incomplete information about carers
- support for young carers, including help at school
- special funding for breaks for carers.

Address for correspondence

Tim Anfilogoff
Department of Health
R211 Wellington House
135–155 Waterloo Road
London SE1 8UG
UK

www.carers.gov.uk

The Care of Older People with Mental Illness: Specialist Services and Medical Training

Reference   Report of a joint working party of the Royal College of Psychiatrists and Royal College of Physicians (1998) *CR69*

Purpose

The main purpose of the report is to provide concerned members of the public with a framework for debate with the commissioners of services for mentally ill older people, and with professional agencies. It covers a wide area, and the text embodies a range of specific recommendations. In particular, attention is drawn to issues in training and research that need to be considered in a strategic response to the needs of an ageing population. The new report updates that published in 1989, but emphasizes that much of what was said then is still relevant. It is noteworthy that old age psychiatry was officially recognized as a specialty within psychiatry within a few months of its publication.

Summary

This is a very influential report published jointly by the Royal College of Physicians and Royal College of Psychiatrists as the result of a joint working party. Its predecessor was published in 1989, and helped to establish recognized standards, advising among other things on the norms for statutory service.

The main recommendations are:

1. By the year 2002 every health district should have a fully resourced specialized service for the psychiatry of old age. The service should be responsive, comprehensive, and provide continuity and quality assurance
2. There should be greater public accountability of commissioners and providers of care for mentally ill older people.
3. Commissioners of services for mentally ill older people should be aware of different service options, have access to appropriate service data, and be ready to learn from examples of good practice.
4. There needs to be a national reference framework against which commissioners and the public can compare practice and standards in their localities. This will require trusts and commissioners to provide service data in the public domain.
5. Specific attention should be paid to particularly vulnerable groups of older people, including the homeless, those with learning disabilities, ethnic and cultural minorities, and older people in institutions or elsewhere who are exposed to the risk of abuse.
6. The health of older people should be designated a key area in revised version of the Health of the Nation and similar initiatives, and within this key area mental health targets should be set.
7. Basic and applied research into mental illness in later life needs to be actively fostered by attention to training, recruitment, resources and removal of impediments.
8. The training requirements of all professionals involved in the care of older people with mental illness should be provided for at undergraduate and postgraduate levels and during professional practice.

Addresses for correspondence

Royal College of Psychiatrists
17 Belgrave Square
London SW1X 8PG
UK

Royal College of Physicians
11 St Andrews Place
London NW1 4LE
UK

A Real Break: A Guidebook for Good Practice in the Provision of Short-Term Breaks as a Support for Care in the Community

Reference   Weightman G (1999) Department of Health

Purpose

Guidance provided to accompany National Carers Strategy, with emphasis on practical arrangements for providing short breaks for carers. This term is preferred rather than 'respite', which is felt to have negative connotations. Several illustrative examples of good practice are provided.

Summary

Some principles of good practice include:

- Where short breaks are provided in long-stay homes, they should be in separate units with their own staff.
- Providing day care in the same site as short breaks has several advantages.
- Specialist short break providers usually offer a variety of activities for users.
- Both those providing and paying for/subsidizing short breaks should take seriously the feedback they receive from users and carers.
- Many schemes provide special training for staff, with users and carers involved in some of this.
- Users and carers are usually involved in some way with planning and management.
- Some schemes enable direct access from users and carers, giving greater flexibility.
- It is useful to have some accommodation for people who want to stay together.
- There are various ways for users and carers to feed back after short breaks, e.g. questionnaires, personal reviews, consultation meetings etc.
- Some schemes keep mementos of short breaks, such as 'holiday' photographs.
- Wherever possible, staff from schemes should visit the user and carer to identify any special needs or resolve any particular anticipatory fears.
- Clarity of purpose – what a break is for – is a hallmark of the best schemes.
- Information packs about available schemes can help users and carers to discover what is on offer and what choices they have.

A good practice checklist is also provided.

Address for correspondence

Tim Anfilogoff
Department of Health
R211 Wellington House
135–155 Waterloo Road
London SE1 8UG
UK

www.doh.gov.uk/pub/docs/doh/realbrea.pdf

Position Statement on Specialist Old Age Psychiatry Team and Nursing and Residential Care Home Residents. Good Practice Principles and Potential Practice Developments

Reference Royal College of Psychiatrists (1998) *Psychiatric Bulletin* 22: 389–90

Purpose

The position statement was produced by the Faculty of Psychiatry of Old Age to address some principles of good practice and potential practice development by specialist old age psychiatry teams in relation to nursing/residential care homes.

Summary

- Specialist teams should assist primary health care teams in maintaining good quality general medical care and support to home residents with particular mental health care needs.
- Specialist teams should be available to assist appropriate needs assessments around entry into homes to enable future care planning and to promote necessary continuity in continuing care.
- Specialist teams should seek good collaborative liaisons with primary care health teams and social services and with geriatric medicine to aid good quality care provision in homes.
- In contact with nursing homes, specialist teams should promote the importance of: (a) approaches to prevention of disability; (b) maintenance of function and a stimulating environment; (c) an ethos of rehabilitation; (d) the need to minimize unnecessary medication; (e) respect for individuality and autonomy; (f) the detection of delirium depression and remedial aspects of dementia.
- Specialist teams should aid continuity of care through their availability for re-referral and ensuring clarity over re-referral and arrangements.
- Specialist teams can promote liaison relationships with primary health care teams through the use of community psychiatric nurses.
- Specialist teams can advise primary health care teams on devising protocols in collaboration with home teams to deal with common problems and good care delivery.
- Specialist teams could advise primary health care teams in homes with joint audit work and good care.
- Specialist teams could explore educational opportunities arising in their contacts with homes and primary health care teams, and be available for education and training programmes.
- Specialist teams could be available to provide purchasers and regulatory authorities with information concerning provision of care by homes.
- Opportunities to implement such principles of good practice will be influenced strongly by resource provision.

Address for correspondence

Dr Rob Jones
Psychiatry of Old Age Faculty
Royal College of Psychiatrists
17 Belgrave Square
London SW1X 8PG
UK

The Interface Between the NHS and the Independent Sector in the Care of Older People with Mental Illness; Recommendations for Improving the Continuity of Care of Older People with Mental Illness

Reference   The Royal College of Psychiatrists (1999) Occasional paper OP45

Purpose

The paper looks at the interface between the NHS and the independent sector with regard to the care and treatment of older people with a mental illness. It reflects the view of the Royal College of Psychiatrists, Faculty of Old Age/Independent Health Care Working Group, and makes specific recommendations about how the quality of care for such people can be improved.

It also recommends group practice guidance on the medical aspects of the discharge of older people with mental illness from hospital to residential and nursing homes.

Summary

Representatives of the Royal College of Psychiatrists and independent providers of care for the elderly should:

- foster good professional relationships and effective and open communications between and within the different professions and providers
- sustain effective collaboration between the FPOA and the independent sector providers of care for older people with mental illness
- work together to improve the quality of care for older people with mental illness on matters of common interest
- identify areas of common agreement which can be jointly supported
- seek to influence government policy on health and social care for older people with mental illness, where appropriate.

Medical

Continuity of medical care would be improved by:

- national standards for discharge from hospitals into the community
- national standards of provision throughout the country for old age psychiatry and CPN input into residential and nursing homes
- national standards for confidentiality and medical records in residential care
- development of specialist GP services to look after residents with mental health problems in the community, whether in residential/nursing homes or in their own home

- national standards for reviewing people with mental health problems in the community – areas such as accommodation needs, drugs and social needs
- national standards in the use and monitoring of psychotropic drugs
- promotion of joint research, both empirical and qualitative, as good practice in the setting of national standards
- national standards for records and reviews in the community.

Nursing

- Robust links are needed between home nursing and care staff and secondary care providers. A good example of how this can be achieved is by joint training sessions.
- To set training standards for care assistants and qualified nurses working with older people with mental health problems.
- To develop tools which are practical and economical in assessing quality of life.
- To agree appropriate standards of accommodation which can be applied nationally for people suffering from dementia and other mental health problems.
- To promote national standards for staffing to care for older people with mental illness in whatever setting.
- To recognize that elderly people with mental health problems often have a multiplicity of needs, both physical and mental.

Social care

- To promote good standards of social activity both on an individual basis and corporately through the care planning process.
- To promote the requirement for individual residents – whether in a residential/nursing home or in the community – to receive individual social care/spiritual care planning as well as corporate activities.
- To recognize the need for adequate day care.
- To promote and facilitate the training of activity organizers or social therapists within the community, both in residential/nursing and in individuals' own homes.
- To encourage the coordination of social activities in a particular area with all providers and voluntary organizations.

- To set good standards of practice in social care.
- To ensure that all staff, including nurses, consider the social care aspects of the care they are delivering.

Safety and the Mental Health Act 1983

- To identify weaknesses in current mental health legislation as it applies to the elderly in both NHS and residential/nursing homes and contribute to the review of the act.
- To give guidance on informed consent.
- To clarify the practical need for safe environments for non-detailed residents.

Patient registration categories

- To recognize the importance of grouping residents according to care needs rather than diagnosis.
- To recognize the need for a flexible and wide variety of appropriate accommodation.
- Development of a nationwide assessment and dependency scoring system.
- To recognize the need for an accepted care planning process for managing individual needs.

Good practice guidance

The following guidance should help to improve the transition to residential care and nursing homes:

- Clinical and personal details should be discussed with the home on a confidential basis. A senior member of staff should always meet the patient before agreeing to the admission.
- A nursing summary and care plan should be transferred to the residential or nursing home with the patient.
- A concise medical discharge summary should be sent to the GP on the date of discharge. It should include physical and psychiatric diagnoses, a brief account of the relevant medical history, a full report of investigations and a comprehensive list of the patient's medication. Ongoing physical and psychiatric problems should be mentioned as well as a clear account of the follow-up arrangements by the multi-disciplinary team. An example of a discharge summary pro forma is provided in the Appendix.

- The residential or nursing home should have a clear procedure for approaching a new GP if this is required. This should allow for the resident or the resident's representative to choose the GP, although in practice this will often be one of the GPs regularly visiting the home. The GP should be identified prior to or at the time of discharge. A patient should not be discharged from hospital unless it is certain that he or she will be accepted on to a GP's list.
- If there is a new GP, relevant medical correspondence – for example, the original psychiatric assessment letters – should be sent to the GP with the discharge summary.
- It should be clear whether the GP wishes correspondence to be sent directly to the surgery or to the residential or nursing home. A residential or nursing home should only receive medical correspondence if there is a satisfactory storage and confidentiality policy for medical notes.
- Active follow-up of patients discharged to residential or nursing home care by a member of the multi-disciplinary team while the patient is settling in to the new environment should be encouraged (preferably within a week of discharge from hospital). Ongoing and unforeseen clinical problems can be dealt with and medication reviewed. The patient should only be discharged from specialist care when he or she is clinically stable and settled into the new environment.
- Special care must be taken for patients moving to a new area. The patient should be referred to the old age psychiatry team within the new area for follow-up, as in the paragraph above. This should only be omitted if there is good reason to be sure that the patient will be clinically stable and specialist follow-up is unnecessary.
- Difficulties with discharge should be fed back to the ward team and can be a useful topic for audit.

Address for correspondence
The Royal College of Psychiatrists
17 Belgrave Square
London SW1X 8PG
UK

Psychological Wellbeing for Users of Dementia Services

Reference British Psychological Society, Division of Clinical Psychology (1994) Briefing Paper No. 2

Purpose

The report was produced by a working party of the Professional Affairs Board of the British Psychological Society in order to produce guidelines for good psychological practice in services for people with dementia. It aims to improve the psychological care for people with dementia by increasing public and professional knowledge and awareness of dementia, making recommendations about the psychological needs of people with dementia and the design and delivery of services for them, and describing methods of service evaluation and quality assurance in the psychological care of people with dementia.

Summary

There are four main sections. The first two discuss definitions, misconceptions about dementia and the principles upon which services should be based. There are then sections on advice to providers and advice to purchasers. There are two appendices, one on psychological approaches to the care of people with dementia.

Advice to providers includes:

1. The basic principle of service provision is the support of people with dementia and their carers in maintaining the lifestyle of their choice.
2. Shared vision. It is essential that all those involved in a dementia service share an agreed understanding and commitment to what the service is trying to achieve.
3. Assessment needs to be comprehensive and should usually take place in the person's own home.
4. Co-ordination requires a care management system involving one person designated to co-ordinate assessment, care planning and review.
5. Relationships. The interaction between the service provider and the service user is the core component of a quality service.
6. Domiciliary services. The main thrust and focus of services should be at the level of the domiciliary workers.
7. Residential care. The aims of residential services should be to ensure the best possible quality of life for people with dementia.
8. Monitoring quality. A checklist of features that should be taken into account in setting standards and auditing the quality of the service is provided.

Advice to purchasers includes:

1. Identification of needs. This includes defining what needs are, identifying the needs of individuals, identifying the needs of communities or populations, prevalence of dementia within the population, studies of the needs of the client group, and other measures at the population level.
2. Vision and objectives of the service. The purchasers' role includes establishing a vision for the service to a particular client group which is shared by all agencies.
3. Contract specifications. Contracts and service-level agreements should be negotiated by the use of aggregated individual needs, together with the outcomes of service delivery, monitored to provide data on unmet needs.
4. Quality and evaluation. Quality specifications should be derived from an understanding of the service objectives, clients' and carers' real needs, their rights, and current legislation including codes of practice and ethical conduct.

Address for correspondence

British Psychological Society
St Andrews House
48 Princess Road East
Leicester LE1 7DR
UK

Chapter 5

Care environments

The Health Care of Older People in Care Homes

Reference   Royal College of Physicians, Royal College of Nursing, British Geriatrics Society (2000)

Purpose

To publish recommendations for the care of older people in nursing and residential homes. It is a joint publication of the Royal College of Physicians, Royal College of Nursing and the British Geriatrics Society.

Summary

Older people in care homes comprise one of the most vulnerable populations in the UK. Their health and care services should be equitable with others and tailored to their specific needs. Yet the organization of such services for care-home residents is haphazard and overshadowed by debates about costs and regulatory mechanisms. The remit of the working party was to explore options for addressing many of the issues that currently prevent older people in care homes from receiving the appropriate level and type of services. The recommendations of the report are intended to build upon and complement policy developments in this area.

Ten statements for action are identified and used to structure the report. Their central theme is to call for an 'integrated interdisciplinary approach' for health and care services for care home residents. Key issues include the need for:

- A standardized interdisciplinary approach to assessment, care planning and care delivery
- Development of the nurse as the lead practitioner in care homes
- Comprehensive systems of service delivery to engage general and specialist aspects of medical practice
- All practitioners engaged in care-home practice to have appropriate education and training
- Relevant programmes of research.

Statements (to become recommendations following discussion at the interdisciplinary workshop)

1. A National Comprehensive Assessment Tool should be adopted that records medical and nursing diagnoses along with disabilities, to enable commissioning, inform care planning and facilitate governance.
2. Individual care planning should clearly address assessed needs and the wishes of the individual. It should also identify expectations, responsibilities and limitations of health and care. The care plan should provide an individual standard from which an individual's progress may be monitored.
3. All the professions and activities that contribute to the care of the individual care home resident should be aligned so as best to meet their needs and preferences. This is most likely to be achieved through a thorough integration of resources.
4. The specialist gerontological nurse should be the lead clinical practitioner for all care-home residents. Definition, recognition, development and training within interdisciplinary care is required.
5. General practitioners need their roles and responsibilities to be defined and supported in care homes. Specific training and qualification and continuing professional development should be encouraged, supported and recognized.
6. There is an urgent need to re-engage specialist geriatric medicine and old age psychiatry in a structured manner to the care-home population.
7. The management of medication and the role of pharmacists could be enhanced by development of their practice to provide total pharmaceutical services to homes rather than individual prescriptions.
8. The organization, application and governance of the professions allied to medicine may be enhanced through integration with other professionals through organization that centres on institutions rather than individuals.
9. Major investment in learning and development is required for medical, nursing and paramedical professions. The concept of a 'teaching nursing home' as a learning organization should be developed.
10. Research is needed to inform further developments that aim to improve health and care outcomes through evidence-based practice for care-home residents.

Address for correspondence

Ms L Parmakis
Royal College of Physicians
11 St Andrew's Place
Regent's Park
London NW1 4LE
UK

Quality Standards for Local Carer Support Services

Reference   www.carers.gov.uk/qualitystan.htm

Purpose

These are carer defined quality standards for local carer support services proposed by a steering group which was set up to agree national standards as part of the implementation of the National Strategy For Carers which have received government approval. The National Strategy for Carers proposed the development of nationally agreed standards:

- to address the current variable quality of local carer support services in order to help and protect individual carers and those for whom they care
- enhance the quality of life for all carers, so no carers are excluded and carers from black and minority ethnic communities are properly included
- assist statutory authorities and other bodies funding carer support services to ensure the service provides an acceptable quality of help to carers

Executive Summary

1. The following standards are based on carers' views of quality and are broadly supported by carers and managers and practitioners from voluntary, health and local authority services who took part in a wide consultation process

2. Many respondents stressed that above all else action is needed by mainstream health, community and social services to deliver good quality support to disabled, ill and frail people. These services also need to recognize and respond to carers better and ensure carers can get help and substitute care in an emergency, a break from caring and night cover.

3. The standards are primarily designed for services exclusively aimed at supporting carers, for example: carer centres, carer support projects, carer groups and services designed to offer carers a break, special help or advice.

4. However, these standards are equally relevant to mainstream health, housing, education, community and social services who will need to address these carer quality standards as well as other quality standards related to the modernization of health and social services and local government.

5. It is recommended that as a pre-requisite for providing a quality service, all carer support services should demonstrate they meet four essential requirements:

- Carers from all local communities are effectively involved in the organization
- The service works in partnership with all local agencies
- The service is clear about its principles, aims and how these will be delivered and monitored
- All staff, including volunteers and trustees, are appropriately trained and supported

6. It is proposed that any service aiming to provide carers with information, a break, emotional support, support to care and maintain carers' own health or support to have a voice will need to meet the relevant standard and accompanying list of conditions

7. The five key standards are:

   (i) Information: any service providing information to carers provides information which is comprehensive, accurate and appropriate, accessible and responsive to individual needs.

   (ii) Providing a break: any service offering a break to carers works in partnership with the carer and person being supported, is flexible and gives confidence and can be trusted.

   (iii) Emotional support: Any service offering emotional support to carers, either on a one-to-one basis or in a group, is sensitive to individual needs, confidential, offers continuity and is accessible to all carers.

   (iv) Support to care and maintain carers' own health: any service which supports carers to care and to maintain their own health and well-being by offering training, health promotion and personal development opportunities is responsive to individual needs

   (v) Having a voice: any service which supports carers to have a voice as an individual and/or collectively is accessible to all carers and is able to act in an independent way.

8. It is proposed these standards for services directed exclusively at carers are monitored through contracting processes. Contracts between the funding organization and the carer support service should include these standards and evidence for meeting each condition obtained systematically as part of the agreement

9. Organizations providing local carer support services should be encouraged to carry out self-audits and

continue to develop their own quality assurance schemes in order to deliver these standards

10. Recommendations from the consultation for action centrally and locally to put these standards into practice include:
    – Support local partnerships between carers, statutory and voluntary organization to address these standards constructively, ensuring no small voluntary or community organization is disadvantaged.
    – Ensure mainstream services meet these quality standards as well as standards for services to the person being supported
    – Support carers to have a key role in monitoring the quality of services
    – Give priority to ensuring carers from all communities are included.

Contact address

Penny Banks
The King's Fund
Chair, Quality Standards Steering Group.
11–13 Cavendish Square
London
W1G 0AN

A Better Home Life: Report of an Advisory Group convened by the Centre for Policy on Ageing

Reference   www.cpa.org.uk/bhl/bhl.htm

Purpose

To produce a code of practice on residential care and to extend it to cover continuing care.

Summary

The code of practice was developed as an update of HOME LIFE which was published in 1984 as the officially commissioned guidance to accompany the registered home act which came into force the following year. The original code was directed to owners and managers of residential care homes and to newly appointed registration and inspection staff in local authority social services departments. The Centre for Policy on Ageing's response is *A Better Home Life* which represents an updated code of practice of the underlying values of respect, dignity, autonomy and fulfilment remain the key underpinnings of the code. The new code is directed exclusively toward old people and deals with their care, not only in residential care homes but also in nursing homes, respite services, continuing care environments and sheltered housing.

The code enshrines the principles of good practice which are

Respect for privacy and dignity
Maintenance of self-esteem
Fostering if independent
Choice and control
Recognition of diversity and individuality
Expression of beliefs
Safety
Responsible risk-taking
Citizen's rights
Sustaining relationships with relatives and friends
Opportunities for leisure activities
High standards of care
Necessary care
Continuity of care
Care which is open to scrutiny

Separate chapters deal with entering care, life in the home, care, management administration and legal issues, staffing, buildings, preventing abuse, dying and death and ensuring standards. Three appendices detail the relevant legislation further reading and useful addresses.

Contact address

Centre for Policy on Ageing
25-31 Ironmonger Row
London EC1V 30P, UK

With Respect to Old Age:
Long-Term Care – Rights and Responsibilities

Reference   **A Report by the Royal Commission on Long-term Care (1999) HMSO**

Purpose

To examine the short- and long-term options for a sustainable system of funding of long-term care for elderly people both in their own homes and in other settings, and within 12 months to recommend how and in what circumstances the cost of such care should be apportioned between public funds and individuals, having regard to:

- the number of people likely to require various kinds of long-term care
- the expectations of elderly people for dignity and security
- the strengths and weaknesses of current arrangements
- fair and efficient ways for individuals to make contributions
- constraints on public funds
- earlier work done by various bodies on this issue.

Summary

Main recommendations:

- The costs of care for those individuals who need it should be split between living costs, housing costs and personal care. Personal care should be available after an assessment, according to need and paid for from general taxation: the rest should be subject to a co-payment according to means.

- The Government should establish a National Care Commission which will monitor longitudinal trends, including demography and spending, ensure transparency and accountability in the system, represent the interests of consumers, encourage innovation, keep under review the market for residential care, nursing care, and set national benchmarks, now and in the future.

Recommendations on funding:

- The Government should ascertain precisely how much money, whether from NHS, Local Authority Social Services and Housing budgets, or from Social Security budgets, goes to supporting older people in residential settings and in people's homes.

- The value of the home should be disregarded for up to 3 months after admission to care in a residential setting (with appropriate safeguards to prevent abuse) and the opportunity for rehabilitation should be included as an integral and initial part of any care assessment before any irreversible decisions on long-term care are taken.

- Measures should be taken to bring about increased efficiency and improved quality in the system, including a more client-centred approach, a single point of contact for the client with devolved budgeting, budgets shared between health, social services and other statutory bodies and greater integration of budgets for aids and adaptations.

- The Commission set out a number of other changes to the current system, such as changing the limits of the means-test, or making nursing care free, which would be of value in themselves, but which would be subsumed by our main recommendation.

- The resources which underpin the Residential Allowance in Income Support should be transferred to local authorities.

- The Government should consider whether 'preserved rights' payments in social security should be brought within the post-1993 system of community care funding, or whether some other solution can be found to address the shortfall in funding experienced by this group.

- The Government's proposals on pooled budgets should be taken further, with pooled budgets being implemented nationally.

- Budgets for aids and adaptations should be included in and accessible from a single budget pool and a scheme should be developed which would enable Local Authorities to make loans for aids and adaptations for individuals with housing assets.

- The system for making direct payments should be extended to the over 65s, subject to proper safeguards and monitoring.

Recommendations on the provision of services:

- Further research on the cost-effectiveness of rehabilitation should be treated as a priority, but this should not prevent the development of a national strategy on rehabilitation led by the Government to be emphasized in the performance framework for the NHS and social services.

- Further longitudinal research is required to track the process and outcomes of preventive interventions and to assess their impact both on quality of life and long-term costs.

- It should be a priority for Government to improve cultural awareness in services offered to black and ethnic minority elders.
- The role of advocacy should be developed locally, with backing from central Government.
- There should be wider consultation on the provision of aids and adaptations and on what should under a new system be free and what should be subject to a charge.

Recommendations on help for carers:

- Better services should be offered to those people who currently have a carer.
- The Government should consider a national carer support package.

Recommendations on information and projections:

- The National Care Commission should be made responsible for making and publishing projections about the overall cost of long-term care at least every 5 years.
- The Government should set up a national survey to provide reliable data to monitor trends in health expectancy.
- The Government should conduct a scrutiny of the shift in resources between various sectors since the early 1980s, and should consider whether there should be a transfer of resources between the NHS and social service budgets given changes in relative responsibilities.
- A more transparent grant and expenditure allocation system should be established. This is a task which could be referred to the National Care Commission.
- Further longitudinal research is required to track the processes and outcomes of preventive interventions and to assess their impact both on quality of life and long-term costs.

Recommendations in relation to younger disabled people:

- In the light of the Commission's main recommendations, the Government should consider how the provision of care according to need would relate to Independent Living Fund provision for the personal care needs of younger disabled people.

Implementing the Commission's recommendations:

- Many of the recommendations can be implemented without the need for primary legislation. Examples include the disregard of housing assets for the first 3 months, changing the means-test limits, or extending the provision of free nursing care. The National Care Commission could be established as a shadow body within Government. The Government is urged to implement the proposals as soon as possible. The need for change is pressing.

The full text of the Commission's report is available on the Royal Commission's website at www.open.gov.uk/royal-commission-elderly/

Crown copyright material is reproduced with the permission of the Controller of Her Majesty's Stationery Office

Address for correspondence

The Stationery Office
The Publications Centre
PO Box 276
London SW8 5DT
UK

With Respect to Old Age

Reference   Royal Commission on Long Term Care
[Addendum – UK Government response]

The UK Government published its response to the Royal Commission report in July 2000, summarized in the NHS Plan (www.nhs.uk/nationalplan/) and given in full under (www.nhs/uk/nationalplan/ltcindex.htm). The Government does not accept that making personal care universally free is the best use of its additional investment on older people's services. It argues that this would not help the least well off, most of whom already have help with the costs of personal care. Instead, NHS nursing care will be provided free in all settings, including nursing homes. The Government also aims to reduce the burden of residential care costs and reduce the need for premature house sales when people enter residential care. There will also be new statutory guidance to reduce variations in charges for care at home.

The Government accepted the Royal Commission's second major recommendation. A National Care Standards Commission will be set up through the Care Standards Act and will begin regulating services in April 2002. The Commission will have four main roles – monitoring, representing the consumer, providing national benchmarks and encouraging the development of better services.

Services for Younger People with Alzheimer's Disease and Other Dementias

Reference   Faculty for the Psychiatry of Old Age, Royal College of Psychiatrists, Council Report number 77 (2000)

Purpose

Policy paper arising from an open forum held by the Faculty in 1996. Old age psychiatrists have always been asked to help in the management of younger patients with dementia, but such requests have probably increased in recent years with reduced numbers of long-stay hospital beds and the emergence of new specific treatments for Alzheimer's disease.

Summary

Recommendations as follows:

1. Purchasing agencies should have specific contractual arrangements for a specialized service for younger patients with AD and other dementias.
2. Each district should have one named consultant responsible for the service, usually an old age psychiatrist. In a population of 500 000, there should be one session for organization and at least one session for clinical input.
3. The number of clinical sessions that will be required depends on the arrangements currently in place, e.g. neuropsychiatry, liaison psychiatry.
4. The early phase of the illness is usually managed by a range of specialists, so coordination and liaison between these and the new dementia service is essential.
5. Easy access to genetic investigation and counselling is important.
6. Collaboration with other specialists, including neurology, neuropsychology, medical genetics, services for learning disabilities, is essential.
7. Areas of particular concern include substance misuse, particularly alcohol; HIV infection; and Creutzfeld-Jakob disease.
8. A population of 500 000 should have a specialist multidisciplinary team.
9. Carers and voluntary organizations should be involved in planning such services.
10. Initial development of services should focus on the organization of diagnostic and community services to provide flexible and individualized care plans.
11. Subsequent developments should include day hospital, respite care and long-stay provision. Separate provision is necessary, as the patients are often physically robust and often do not integrate easily with frail older people.
12. Recommendations to be audited in 2001 by the Alzheimer's Society and the Faculty for Psychiatry of Old Age.

Additional references

Allen H, Baldwin R (1995) The referral, investigation and diagnosis of presenile dementia: two services compared. *International Journal of Geriatric Psychiatry* **10**: 185–90.

Alzheimer's Disease Society (1996) *Younger People with Dementia: A Review and Strategy.*

Newens AJ, Forster DP, Kay DWK *et al* (1993) Clinically diagnosed presenile dementia of the Alzheimer type in the Northern Health Region: ascertainment, prevalence, incidence and survival. *Psychological Medicine* **23**: 631–44.

Address for correspondence

Book Sales Office
Royal College of Psychiatrists
17 Belgrave Square
London SW1X 8PG
UK

www.rcpsych.ac.uk

Ready to Go Home. Rehabilitation Re-discovered

Reference   Age Concern Policy Unit (1999) *Ready to go Home. Rehabilitation Re-discovered.* ISBN 0-86242-307-4

Purpose

To underscore the benefits of rehabilitation overcoming current difficulties in relation to treatment of older people in hospital.

Summary

An ageing population is the reality of life in our nation. The demographic facts are clear. Given a fair wind, most adults will live to be old. In the next millennium, the reality of day-to-day life will be an increasing number of older people; the number of pensioners aged 65 and over will increase, but more importantly those in the oldest age groups will show a proportionally greater increase. Today's NHS is struggling to cope: nowhere is this more true than in relation to older people. Certainly, the present structural organization of health and social care systems could not be stretched to meet the future needs of the increased elderly population. Consequently, a great deal more work is needed, if appropriate services for older people are to be developed. These should include:

- The setting of standards and monitoring of performance to ensure high quality service provisions
- Acknowledging the proportion of older people occupying hospital beds, and ensuring training of all hospital staff who may be involved in caring for them
- Ending the practice of using older people as scapegoats for problems which have arisen consequent upon the historic errors of planners.
- Providing appropriately staffed and equipped facilities to ensure all older people have the benefits of time to recover, and to undergo a rehabilitation programme in order to avoid 'warehousing' at home or in homes
- Providing good quality hospital services during and after holiday periods
- Admitting to care homes only when a rehabilitation programme would not enable supported living at home
- Holding to account for the oversight of their care, the multidisciplinary team who decided that an older person needs institutional care
- Recognizing that failure to provide comprehensive, knowledge-based care for the current generation of older people will eventually disadvantage ourselves.

Address for correspondence

Professor Peter H Millard
Eleanor Peel Professor of Geriatric Medicine
Department of Geriatric Medicine
St George's Hospital Medical School
Cranmer Terrace
London SW17 0RE
UK

The Assessment of Frail Elderly People Being Considered for or in Receipt of Continuing Care: A Joint Policy Statement

Reference   British Geriatrics Society, Association of Directors of Social Services and Royal College of Nursing (1995)

Purpose

This statement is aimed at those committed to commissioning and providing the best quality of health care for older people. It argues that the key to both the most effective patient outcome and maximizing cost savings is informed, multidisciplinary assessment.

Summary

1. Multidisciplinary assessment must include expert medical and nursing assessment to ensure:
    *   accurate diagnoses
    *   appropriate functionally-orientated treatment
    *   assessment of potential for rehabilitation
    *   appropriate identification of services required.
2. More involvement of primary care teams is required, both as purchasers and providers of care.
3. Medical inputs into nursing and residential homes should be delivered by those who have specialist knowledge, skill and training in the health care of old age.
4. Older people, wherever they reside, require the services of a properly trained multidisciplinary workforce.
5. This requires the Government to give priority to targets which identify high quality treatment outcomes to older people in the community and in hospitals.
6. Specialists in the medicine and health of old age have a vital role, in conjunction with local authority social services departments, in making a reality of community care.
7. Most frail older people, given a choice, prefer high quality hospital short-term care followed by a return to their own homes in the community. The document calls upon the Government and the NHS to give the highest priority to the engagement of trained and skilled practitioners in assessment for care and treatment that enables and ultimately empowers older people as citizens.

Addresses for correspondence

Dr Alistair Main
Chair, Policy Committee
BGS
Queen Elizabeth Medical Centre
Edgbaston
Birmingham B15 2TH
UK

Martin Shreeve
Chair, ADSS Services for Elderly People Committee
Social Services Dept
Civic Centre
Wolverhampton WV1 1RT
UK

Pauline Ford
Nursing Advisor for Older People
RCN
20 Cavendish Square
London W1M 0AB
UK

The Transfer of Frail Older NHS Patients to Other Long-Stay Settings

Reference National Health Service Executive (1998) Health Service Circular HSC 1998/048. Department of Health

Purpose

This is an official circular providing guidance in response to public concern about transfers of frail old people from NHS settings, usually following the closure of old hospitals or long-stay wards. The aim is to ensure the safe transfer of patients to more suitable settings where they will continue to receive quality health care.

Summary

The guidance covers:

- consultation
- the project plan
- the needs of the individual and their relatives or carers
- the process of transfer and the role of the receiving setting
- arrangements for follow-up and monitoring.

To help in the planning and implementation process, action checklists are provided for each topic.

Address for correspondence

Copies available from:
Department of Health
PO Box 410
Wetherby LS23 7LL
UK

www.open.gov.uk/doh/outlook/htm

No Accounting for Health. Health Commissioning for Dementia

Reference   Alzheimer's Disease Society (1997)

Purpose

The report was commissioned to examine the effect of delegating the commissioning of services for people with dementia to Local Health Authorities, and to specifically assess whether the money had followed the patient.

Summary

1. *Lack of assessment.* Of the health authorities, 485 had not carried out an assessment of the needs of people with dementia in their area.
2. *Inconsistent approach.* There is no consistent approach by health authorities to assessing the needs of people with dementia in their area.
3. *Lack of consultation with GPs.* Of the health authorities that carried out an assessment of need, 72% had not involved GPs in this work – despite their role in early diagnosis and assessment of dementia.
4. *Lack of consultation with carers.* Of health authorities that carried out an assessment of local needs, 53% did not involve carers.
5. *Resources not identified.* Seventy-nine per cent of health authorities were unable to identify the resources spent on dementia care in the current financial year.
6. *Needs not reflected in budgets.* Of health authorities that had carried out a needs assessment, 73% could not then identify resources allocated to dementia services.
7. *Variable spending.* Spending per person with dementia can range from approximately £600 to £1800 per year, depending on the health authority in which they live.
8. *Spending not identified.* Fifty per cent of health authorities did not give an answer or were unable to provide information about how much they spent on dementia care in the last 3 years.
9. *Spending freeze.* Of health authorities which expressed an opinion, 19% said their future spending on dementia care would 'remain stable'.
10. *Poor budget control.* Health authorities are failing to ensure appropriate and rational allocation of resources, equality of access and budgeting control – key functions of a commissioning body in the health service.

Recommendations

To the government

The Department of Health should issue urgent guidance on how health authorities ought to assess the current and future needs of people with dementia and their carers.

The Department of Health should make the assessment of the needs of people with dementia one of the key priorities for health authorities in the coming year.

The Department of Health should ensure equality of access to health care and treatment in the National Health Service for people by introducing:

– national eligibility criteria for long-term care
– national standards for community care
– a national protocol for access to new diagnostic tests and treatments for Alzheimer's disease.

The Department of Health should review priority setting and expenditure plans in the health service for delivering services to people with dementia and their carers.

To health authorities

Directors of public health should lead the co-ordination of assessment of local needs of people with dementia.

Health authorities should establish dementia care management units which will assume organizational responsibility for the planning and provision of services to meet the needs of people with dementia and their carers, regardless of their age.

Address for correspondence

Alzheimer's Society
Gordon House
10 Greencoat Place
London SW1P 1PH
UK

Nursing Home Placements for Older People in England and Wales: A National Audit 1995–1998

Reference   Pulford C, Millard P (1999) Out of sight. *General Medicine* 13–14. ISBN Number: 0 9535208 0 3

Purpose

A Report Commissioned by the Clinical Audit Unit of the National Health Service in England and Wales

Summary

In 1995, an audit commissioned by the South East London Health Commissioning Agency (*The Right Person, The Right Time, The Right Place*, 1995) involved a sample of 157 elderly residents in 25 nursing homes. Judging by Barthel scores, 35% of these residents were found to have care needs below the level expected for nursing home residents. The audit also found a serious lack of documentation in nursing homes, making it difficult to determine the reason for nursing home placement or the changing needs of the residents after placement.

A larger audit was commissioned by the NHS Executive to discover whether the problems observed in South East London were also apparent nationwide. In 1995/1996, centrally trained, locally recruited audit teams collected data in six areas: Birmingham, Exeter, Ipswich, Newcastle, Swansea and London (Merton, Sutton and Wandsworth). Data were collected on 897 older people in 150 nursing homes. Following local feedback of audit results, a sample of nursing homes in each area was re-audited to determine whether suitability for placement and the quality of documentation had improved. The second audit involved a sample of 282 older people in 40 nursing homes.

Nursing home matrons often differed from the audit teams in their assessment of need. The matrons considered that 93% of residents were appropriately placed. However, based on Barthel scores, the national audits suggested 28% were less dependent than might be expected. Among those judged less dependent than might be expected among nursing home residents, 18% had dementia as first admission diagnosis. The national audit showed that at least one-third of nursing home residents had improved Barthel scores since they were first admitted. Fifty per cent of residents with lesser care needs (Barthel score greater than 10) had improved since admission. The auditors considered that 17% no longer needed nursing care. This suggests that the decision to admit to permanent nursing home care may have been made too soon, i.e. before rehabilitation was completed.

The national audits found medical and social work documentation on admission was poor among 59% and 40%, respectively, of nursing home residents. Eighty per cent of older people admitted from hospital (836 people) had some nursing documentation, compared with 50% of the 318 people admitted from their own homes. Involvement of either a consultant geriatrician or psycho-geriatrician was recorded as having taken place for 58% of older people admitted from hospital, and 6% admitted directly from their own homes. Fifty-six per cent of the residents' medical notes were kept in the doctor's surgery and not in the nursing home.

Results from the second national audit showed that among the subset of nursing home residents sampled, adequacy of documentation had improved. For instance, adequacy of medical documentation improved from 37% to 67%, social worker documentation from 21% to 61% and nursing documentation from 39% to 67%. Apparent appropriateness of placement had minimally improved from 84% to 86%. These improvements may have been in part due to the work of local audit teams.

This study suggests there is a national problem concerning the adequacy of rehabilitation before nursing home admission, and the adequacy of medical, nursing and social work documentation relating to residents on admission. Regular, local audit is needed to ensure that older people are not simply warehoused in nursing homes.

Address for correspondence

Department of Geriatric Medicine
St George's Hospital Medical School
Cranmer Terrace
London SW17 0RE
UK

Service Standards for the NHS Care of Older People

Reference   A Health Services Accreditation Publication sponsored by the Centre for Policy on Ageing (1999)
ISBN 1 901097 45 5

Purpose

To assess standards of health services for older people, and related issues, and of relevant social care.

Summary

Section 1   Outlines the context for delivery of services to older people; indicates the scope of the report and the principles that should govern the provision of care.

Section 2   Examines health and social care available in the community, including the organization and delivery of services, access, standards for home visits, assessment and care planning. The report focuses on the need for multi-professional integrated joint service team work. Standards for risk management, health and safety and health promotion are also included.

Section 3   Introduces standards for the care of the older person when presenting at A&E, on admission, and as an inpatient. Particular issues such as pain management, nutrition, ward facilities and staffing are among those examined. The section also sets standards for outpatient services, day hospital and rehabilitation services. The importance of multidisciplinary cross-boundary team work is stressed throughout.

Section 4   Concentrates on the need for applied communication policies which link patients, carers, primary and secondary care and social care agencies. Topics addressed include referral practice, record keeping, and discharge (transfer of care) communication. The role of carers is emphasized, and standards are recommended for a Hospital at Home scheme.

Section 5   Deals with consent, confidentiality, privacy and dignity, and complaints procedures. The impact of these issues on the patient's view of the NHS is emphasized. Particular needs of members of ethnic groups are examined. Guidance for action on suspected elder abuse, both domestic and institutional, is given. Key features of care of the terminally ill are covered.

Section 6   Looks at strategies for preventing avoidable falls by older people, both within the community and in the acute care environment.

Section 7   This section looks at the incidence and pathology of dementia. It examines the management of dementia in the community and in the acute sector. Strategies are proposed to increase true awareness of the condition and to manage its treatment and/or the care of patients with a dementia syndrome.

Section 8   The management of patients with stroke serves as a valid proxy for the care of the older person, raising questions of the application of evidence-based practice, the necessity for clear quality standards applying to inpatient care, discharge and follow-up/rehabilitation, and the clinical audit of services delivered. Each aspect is considered, and standards which define safe and effective care are specified.

Section 9   Section 9 introduces and explains the importance of routine, systematic clinical multi-professional audit of the delivery of care to older persons. It sets out standards for the organization and management of audit programmes and key topics which should feature in the audit of care provided in the acute and community sectors.

Addresses for correspondence

Centre for Policy on Ageing
25–31 Ironmongers Row
London EC1V 3QP
UK

cpa@cpa.org.uk

Health Services Accreditation
Rutherford Park
Marley Lane
Battle
East Sussex TN33 0EZ
UK

info@nhs-accreditation.co.uk

www.nhs-accreditation.co.uk

Fit for the Future? National Required Standards for Residential and Nursing Homes for Older People

Reference   Department of Health (1999)

Purpose

The document outlines the Government's commitment to national standards and describes how the Centre for Policy on Aging was commissioned to produce nationally required standards. It sets out the context in which national standards would operate, and highlights some of the issues in which implementation might arise. It invites comments on these standards and on suggestions made for a smooth transition to their introduction.

Summary

The standards are presented in great detail under eleven main headings, each with sub-topics, a note of relevant legislation and existing regulations, the national required standard, the evidence for this standard and the outcome of it.

The standards are:

1. *The home's brochure and prospectus*
    1.1   The brochure and prospectus
    1.2   Aims and objectives
    1.3   Aims into practice
    1.4   Contractual details
    1.5   Facilities and services
    1.6   Accuracy
    1.7   Registration certificate
2. *Rights of individual residents*
    2.1   Respect
    2.2   Privacy
    2.3   Terms of address
    2.4   Risk taking
    2.5   Civil rights
    2.6   Choice
    2.7   Advocacy
    2.8   Personal property
    2.9   Access to records
3. *Complaints*
    3.1   Procedure
    3.2   Records
    3.3   Staff
4. *Policies, procedures, records and protocols*
    4.1   Records
    4.2   Prevention of abuse
    4.3   Restraint
    4.4   Infection control

    4.5   Fire safety
    4.6   Health and safety
    4.7   Food safety
    4.8   Medicines
    4.9   Nutrition
    4.10   Other policies and procedures
5. *Health and personal care*
    5.1   Assessment
    5.2   Care
    5.3   The care plan
    5.4   Case notes
    5.5   Personal care
    5.6   Medication
    5.7   Care from external agencies
6. *Daily life and social activities*
    6.1   The organization of daily life
    6.2   Consultation
    6.3   Social activities
    6.4   Supporters, visitors
    6.5   Links with the local community
    6.6   Involvement of volunteers
7. *Food preparation, meals and mealtimes*
    7.1   Food policy
    7.2   Residents' food
    7.3   Menus
    7.4   Mealtimes
    7.5   Food purchase, storage and preparation
8. *Dying and death*
    8.1   Policy and procedures
    8.2   Information about the resident
    8.3   Care of people who are dying
    8.4   Supporters' involvement
    8.5   Place of dying
    8.6   Payment of fees on death of a resident
    8.7   Notification of death
9. *The physical environment*
    9.1   Location
    9.2   Overall style and philosophy
    9.3   State of repair
    9.4   General design
    9.5   Toilets in communal areas
    9.6   Residents' room size
    9.7   Shared accommodation
    9.8   Baths
    9.9   En suite facilities

Address for correspondence

Dept of Health

PO Box 777

London SE1 6XH

UK

Older People with Mental Health Problems Living Alone: Anyone's Priority?

Reference   Barnes, D (1997) Social Services Inspectorate and Department of Health

Purpose

The need is to highlight the particular issues raised by the care of older people with mental health problems who live alone, and the aim of the report is to stimulate thinking on policy and the planning of services for older people in this group. It is neither a guidance document nor a research report, and reports issues, dilemmas and ideas found in the community care response to the particular needs of this care group.

A workshop was held to which staff from Health, Social Services and the independent sector were invited to expose some of the main issues and following this a Social Services Inspectorate study team visited four local authorities.

Summary

1. The findings in this report did not stem from an SSI inspection, nor were they the outcome of systematic research, but were the result of discussions held in workshops, working group meetings and during visits to four local authorities. The visits were limited in number and time, and the SSI Study Team concentrated their enquiries on a small range of issues. This is perhaps why the results tend to ask more questions than they answer, but it was never intended that firm conclusions would be drawn from this study. Instead, the report poses tentative findings which agencies might be interested in taking into account when planning, purchasing and providing a service for older people with mental health problems who live alone.

2. Older mentally ill people who live alone are an important group of users of community care. They are a significantly large group, and their number is rising. They can also be very dependent on services to support their wish, or need, to live at home on their own. Their care can therefore be expensive. Consequently, services must make the best use of resources, ensuring that the older person's needs are being understood and met in the most effective way.

3. Older people with mental illness who live alone are also a very diverse group in terms of their background, life histories and circumstances, as well as their mental and physical health. Their situation is often liable to rapid change, and can result in them being a risk to themselves and others. For all these reasons, they present a challenge to community care. They need access to a very wide range of health and social services and, like other older people, they need appropriate housing, adequate income and security. In addition, they are particularly vulnerable because of their mental illness, and may need protection.

4. During the study visits, stress was placed on the importance of joint work between health and social services so that an integrated service is delivered to the older person. Like books supported by bookends, the care of an older mentally ill person alone can collapse if either side of the support is missing. To maintain this support, a flexible response from both types of services was felt to be crucial.

5. In order to allocate resources and plan strategically for this group, it was recognized that better information was required. It was suggested that some improvement could be achieved quickly by collating information currently collected by agencies for different purposes, but only by knowing more about the size and needs of this group could their profile be raised and appropriate, good quality care planned for.

6. The complexity of assessing the needs of older people with mental illness living alone was emphasized. Each individual must first be assessed as a person, secondly as an older person and thirdly as someone with mental health problems. This could not be done in a day. It took skill and understanding if it was to be done sensitively, and a system was required to make sure that it was carried out by the most appropriate person.

7. The need for a flexible response from services was highlighted. Older mentally ill people are not going to conform to the needs of the service – the service must respond to them. Packages of care for this group were found to be becoming more personalized, and more able to adjust to constant change and sudden crisis. Innovative and imaginative specialist mental health services were found to be particularly responsive. Access to advocates to help older people exert their rights and express their views was widely valued.

8. Services which were often found to be undervalued were domiciliary support services and home care. Although they provided a crucial element in enabling older people with mental illness to stay at home, workers were not always given the opportunity to give

feedback into client reviews and some felt unable to use their judgement in responding to older people's needs.

9. Emphasis was constantly placed on the importance of co-ordinating the care of older people with mental illness who live alone. They may not have any family to contribute to this and their lives can often be chaotic. Therefore, it was considered essential for someone to take responsibility for arranging, monitoring and reviewing care packages. In straightforward cases it was sometimes felt to be appropriate for a service provider or a relative to act as co-ordinator, but in more complex cases this should be done by a care manager.

10. The need for specialist skills and knowledge for the care of mentally ill elders was a key theme throughout the study's findings and was regarded as important in every aspect of care, including assessment, acceptance of risk, providing service and protection. Therefore training is vital and should be undertaken jointly across agencies wherever possible.

11. In concentrating on older people with mental health problems who live alone, the study identified marginalization of this group, and yet found a battery of policies and examples of good practice which were highly applicable to them. There were also signs of change. Carers are stressing the issues and making demands. More documentation and information is becoming available, helping to raise awareness that this is a growing group of people who require a specialist community care response. Through more joint work with social care, health and housing agencies, perhaps we are working towards a position where an answer can be given to the question, 'Whose priority are older people with mental health problems who live alone?'. They are a priority for everybody.

Address for correspondence

Department of Health
PO Box 410
Wetherby LS23 7LN
UK

Family Involvement in Care for Persons with Dementia

Reference   University of Iowa Gerontological Nursing Interventions Research Center, Research Dissemination Core (1999) University of Iowa

Purpose

To provide guidelines for implementing a program to involve family members in the care of their relatives with dementia and to assist family members to enact meaningful and satisfactory caregiving roles regardless of the setting. The guidelines are intended for nurses and nurse practitioners and were developed through expert consensus using all available source documents on the subject.

Summary

The guideline recommends orientation of family members to the physical care environments, to foster an awareness of the environmental assets as well as the potential deficits; the education of all caregivers on negotiation and formation of a partnership agreement; and the education of family members involved in care. The guideline recognizes the difficulties that many family caregivers have when the patient with dementia must adapt to a new care situation, and provides a framework whereby family caregivers can be involved in the caregiving process in this new care setting.

Address for correspondence

University of Iowa Gerontological Nursing Interventions Research Center
Research Dissemination Core
4118 Westlawn
Iowa City, IA 52242-1100
USA

Experiences of Care in Residential and Nursing Homes: A Survey

Reference   Alzheimer Disease Society (1997)

Purpose

Postal survey of carers and former carers belonging to Alzheimer's Disease Society (covering England, Wales and Northern Ireland), asking about the type of home occupied by a person with dementia, quality of care, attitudes of staff and professionals, and particular examples of mistreatment or neglect; 1421 completed questionnaires were received.

Summary

1. Ten per cent of carers cited cases of mistreatment or neglect.
2. Over half (56%) were not consulted over use of drugs in the person's management.
3. Many carers gave poor or average ratings for personal care, continence management and occupational therapy.
4. Almost half felt that support from doctors was poor or average.
5. Forty-four per cent felt they had inadequate information, and one in five were not consulted about the person's care.
6. Deterioration in carer's health was the commonest reason for the person with dementia to enter a home.
7. Eighty-five per cent of respondents said care provided by homes was satisfactory.
8. Over 70% rated food, staff attitudes and physical environment highly.

Recommendations

Residential and nursing homes and the associations running them should address the need for improved standards of care for people with dementia, including:

- better communication and consultation with relatives
- reduction in drugs to control behaviour
- active strategies for incontinence prevention or incontinence management
- active strategy for safe wandering
- programme of purposeful and relevant activities for residents
- improved health care and more effective involvement of GPs
- clear and effective complaints procedure
- regular training for all care workers.

Government should:

- consider a single registration system for care homes to allow extra care as people's needs change
- extend present system of lay inspectors to include nursing homes and actively involve carers
- encourage training initiatives to raise skill levels among care staff
- issue new guidance on use of neuroleptics in managing people with dementia
- improve the medical supervision of care homes.

The Alzheimer's Disease Society should:

- in partnership with other organizations, improve and make more accessible the information given to families to assist in the difficult task of selecting a care home
- continue to develop its Care Learning Programme for care workers in homes, and seek to encourage improved training for dementia care.

Address for correspondence

Alzheimer's Society
Gordon House
10 Greencoat Place
London SW1P 1PH
UK

www.alzheimers.org.uk

They Look After Their Own Don't They? Inspection of Community Care Services for Black and Ethnic Minority Older People

Reference   Social Care Group, Department of Health and Social Services Inspectorate (1998)

Purpose

The report summarizes a survey of an inspection to evaluate the extent to which Social Services Departments' arrangements for planning and delivering community care services appropriately address the needs of ethnic minority older people. The fieldwork was conducted in eight local authority areas which each had a significant ethnic minority group.

Description

Policies, strategies and planning

In order to overcome institutional racism, SSDs should re-think the approach of providing a common service for everyone and treating both black and white older people the same. This requires greater confidence in developing targeted and specific services, rather than being over concerned that this means special treatment for black elders. SSDs should overcome discriminatory institutional barriers to services for ethnic minority older people by establishing inclusive consultation arrangements and other equality practices.

Elected members and senior managers should have explicit policies and strategies, and should not rely on committed people within the organization to promote and develop the equality services for service users and carers. Race issues should be incorporated into community care policies and strategies. These should take full account of the political, social and economic discrimination faced by black elders, rather than marginalizing their needs. Effective joint planning between agencies for black elders must be based on a common understanding of local ethnic minority communities, and include them in the process. The planning process should be informed by effective management information systems which support data collection about the needs of black elders. Ethnic record-keeping and monitoring must be developed to ensure that SSDs can analyse referrals, assessments and service information. They should be capable of identifying service deficits and influencing service planning for black elders.

Communication and information

Information about services and rights provides service users and carers with an important safeguard against racism,

abuse and discrimination. SSDs need to develop, with ethnic minority communities, strategies for communication and information which are more innovative and ensure that information reaches black elders inaccessible formats. SSDs need to ensure that clear protocols and guidelines on the use of interpreters and translation, and training on how to make effective use of these resources. These arrangements should be monitored.

Assessment, care management and review

Assessors play a critical role in ensuring equality of access to services and need to:

- develop antidiscriminatory practice, cultural sensitivity and skills in empowering service users and their carers throughout the assessment process
- be aware of their own knowledge and skill limitations in this area of work, and know when it is appropriate to involve someone else with more specific expertise
- be informed and flexible and avoid seeing black elders as problems, or blaming individuals who do not 'fit' into existing inappropriate services
- learn from the life experiences of ethnic minority older people, and fashion services to meet their needs.

Joint arrangements for multi-agency and multidisciplinary assessment and care management processes for black elders should be improved for the benefit of black elders.

Service delivery

The needs of black elders are the same as those of other people, but sometimes these needs should be met in specific and different ways. The commitments and priorities for black elders proclaimed in Community Care Plans and other strategy documents should be capable of implementation by front-line staff with confidence. SSDs should stimulate the development of services both in-house and within the independent sector to provide a range of appropriate residential, domiciliary and day-care services for black elders. SSD should have mechanisms to establish the suitability, appropriateness and effectiveness of the services delivered. Complaints procedures should be available to black elders in appropriate local languages and formats. Ethnic monitoring of all complaints should be introduced which take account of specific complaints about discrimination, abuse and harassment.

Protection from abuse

The generic elder abuse policies and procedures should be further developed with other agencies and ethnic minority groups to address the experiences of black elders, who may suffer racial abuse and harassment.

Staff vary in their level of understanding and interest, and there should be training strategies targeted at those who work directly with ethnic minority older people to develop their skills further. SSDs should have race equality policies and procedures, and ensure that all staff are acquainted with these.

Address for correspondence

Department of Health
PO Box 777
London SE1 6XH
UK

Alzheimer's Disease and Chronic Dementing Illnesses

Reference   University of Iowa Gerontological Nursing Interventions Research Center, Research Dissemination Core (1995) University of Iowa

Purpose

To present interventions and activities designed to minimize secondary symptom presentation in patients with Alzheimer's disease and related disorders. The guideline is directed towards nurse and nurse practitioners.

Summary

Interventions are identified which can be used to increase the functional quality of life for patients at risk with problems related to dementia. These include using rest periods at least twice a day, minimizing changes in their environment and promoting consistency, reducing misleading and inappropriate stimuli in the environment, ensuring safety, and encouraging appropriate fluid and nutritional balance.

Address for correspondence

University of Iowa Gerontological Nursing Interventions
Research Center
Research Dissemination Core
4118 Westlawn
Iowa City, IA 52242-1100
USA

www.nursing.uiowa.edu/gnirc

The Cornerstone of Care:
Inspection of Care Planning for Older People

Reference   Social Care Group, Department of Health and Social Services Inspectorate (1997)

Purpose

The aim of the inspection was to assess Social Services Departments' capacity to respond appropriately to the needs of older people who live alone in the community or with carers.

Summary

The report produces the findings of inspections in seven local authorities.

Responsive services

SSDs should endeavour to make services responsive to the varied needs of older people and their carers. This requires flexible services able to meet a range of circumstances, including in some instances the provision of help with cleaning and household maintenance. The ongoing development of care management skills and practice is essential if systems are to be used effectively and older people's potential is to be realized. SSDs, in conjunction with housing authorities, must do more to speed up housing adaptations and prevent unnecessary dependence on care services.

Care planning

SSDs should differentiate between the coordinating and intensive types of care management. They should ensure that the latter is limited to those people who need it. Decisions about the skills of staff to be deployed and about monitoring and reviewing arrangements should reflect this. Unnecessary duplication of assessment processes should be avoided. Care plans appropriate to the complexity of individual circumstances should be drawn up for users in receipt of services. Wherever possible, the emphasis should be on simplicity and clarity. SSI's *Care Management and Assessment: Practitioners Guide* (1991) (HMSO) contains useful advice on what individual care plans might include.

Participation

Continued efforts are needed to promote the involvement of older people and their carers in the care planning process. Further impetus is required if the provisions of the Carers (Recognition and Services) Act 1995 are to be realized and service providers are to make practical support for carers a high priority. The Department of Health's Policy Guidance and Practice Guide (LAC(96)7-HSG(96)8) are of help here. SSDs should promote the development of advocacy services and access to them by older people and their carers.

Information and communication

Potential users and carers and relevant health, social services and other professionals should be properly informed by SSDs about the range of services available, how to access them, and any eligibility criteria or charging policies which may apply.

Equal opportunities

SSDs and others should develop an approach to the care of older people which challenges commonly held assumptions about the inevitability of disability and dependence, and builds upon strengths and support networks. Service take-up by black and minority ethnic communities should be measured, and SSDs should use this information in the development of appropriate services. Assessors need to be aware of the relevance of sensory impairment in older people, and ensure appropriate health examination and support.

Address for correspondence

Department of Health
PO Box 410
Wetherby LS23 7LN
UK

High Quality Long-Term Care for Elderly People: Guidelines and Audit Measures

Reference   Royal College of Physicians and British Geriatrics Society (1992)

Purpose

The report contains guidelines on the management of common challenges encountered in long-term care, implementation of which would enhance its quality. The report refers to the care of elderly people who have been designated as permanent hospital residents. The Royal College of Physicians and the British Geriatric Society wish to signal their continued interest in the quality of life and care enjoyed by elderly people in long-term care.

Summary

The report contains over 100 references. The eight guidelines described are:

1. Preserving autonomy
2. Promoting urinary continence
3. Promoting faecal continence
4. Optimizing drug use
5. Managing falls and accidents
6. Preventing pressure sores
7. Optimizing the environment, equipment and aids
8. The medical role in long-term care.

Conclusions

The recommendations of this report owe much to the consensus of interested and experienced specialists, as there is a paucity of data on which to base firm conclusions. The impact that the guidelines, and the Royal College of

Physicians CARE scheme, may have on the quality of care cannot be predicted with certainty. However, the numerous descriptions of very poor standards of long-term care would suggest that adoption of the very basic measures set out in this document may transform the care received by many residents.

The guidelines and the CARE package derived from them will need to be refined with use. Our aim must be to obtain a uniform quality of excellence in long-term care for elderly people, and to this end a uniform approach is essential. We suggest, therefore, that all health and local authorities adopt these guidelines and the CARE scheme.

In addition, a number of areas for future clinical, quality assurance and health service research have been highlighted by the preparation of this report. Fertile areas include the prevalence of key indicator problems, evaluation of long-term care entry panels, care plan implementation, the comparative effect of improved environments and the CARE scheme, and the assessment of resident satisfaction. Above all, an authoritative review of the staffing and other resources needed for good quality long-term care is urgently needed.

Address for correspondence

Royal College of Physicians
9 Queen Square
Edinburgh EH2 1JQ
UK

At Home with Dementia: Inspection of Services for Older People with Dementia in the Community

Reference   Social Services Inspectorate (1996) Department of Health

Purpose

To evaluate arrangements and services provided by local authorities to maintain older people in the community, including home support, day care and short breaks. An inspection of social services for older people with dementia in the community in eight local authorities was conducted.

Summary

Service delivery

- The best practice appeared to occur where there were good collaborative arrangements between SSD and NHS staff who were content to blur the boundaries of their activities, but such arrangements were sometimes under threat because of pressure to define boundaries more clearly and to determine the costs of health and social care.
- The commitment, knowledge and skill of many practitioner staff was high.
- Most service users remained dependent on traditional services but some innovative practice was witnessed which was beginning to address a needs-led approach.
- The major growth of independently provided home care in most LAs was often providing more choice and flexibility. But there was cause for anxiety about the standards of practice in some independent agencies, about alleged unreliability of some provision, and about the unhelpful impact on this group of service users when they were expected to cope with home care from more than one source.
- Services were mostly provided for older people generally, and varied in quality from very good to quite poor, even within the same authority. Where specialist services had been provided, or there were good collaborative arrangements between providers from different agencies, or particular thought given to how best to provide for older people with dementia within a generic service, the services were noticeably better. Older people who did not have dementia often found the presence and behaviour of older people with dementia in day and residential care distressing.
- Transport arrangements sometimes undermined the potential value of some services for older people with dementia, most usually because of their failure to respond to the needs of individual users and carers.
- Carers were almost universal in their praise for the services they received and the staff who delivered them.

Strategies and plans

- Most SSDs were struggling, and sometimes failing, to work jointly with the NHS locally around strategic and planning issues, despite the fact that most SSD and NHS staff reported good working relationships with each other.
- It was the major complaint of the carers that little of the information which SSDs made available about their community care provision was specific to the needs of older people with dementia, as distinct from older people generally.

Assessment and care planning

- The quality of collaborative working arrangements on assessment, care management and service delivery at practitioner level were generally good where they existed.
- Collaborative work at practitioner level involved SSD staff, nurses and consultants together with members of the primary health care team, though not usually GPs.
- The over-75 health check had not initiated any referrals to SSDs in the cases surveyed.
- The implementation of the Care Programme Approach with this client group was extremely patchy, and seemed to depend partly on whether services were provided primarily as part of services for older people or as part of mental health services.
- Despite statutory requirement and guidance, the copying of care plans to service users and carers was a rarity.

Monitoring and review

- Monitoring of service delivery was completed very patchily, and in some cases not very adequately. In some SSDs monitoring was left to providers to carry out themselves.
- High quality, timely review of care plans involving service users and their carers in the process was quite rare. Some authorities were committed to the concept but had difficulty in delivering to reasonable time scales.

Assessment and management of risk taking

- Most practitioner staff were routinely considering issues of risk management for this group of service users, but in only one SSD were they supported by explicit policies which set out what the LA's expectations were and supported staff in this area of work.

Protection from abuse
- Half the SSDs had a policy on elder abuse, but only two of these were joint with other agencies.

Equality of opportunity
- Practice on equality of opportunity was encouraging insofar as it was concerned with meeting cultural needs. Gender needs were poorly served by home care services, which could rarely meet the need for care by male staff when this was required.

Crown copyright is reproduced with the permission of the Controller of Her Majesty's Stationery Office

Appendix 1

Which Guidelines to Use and When*

To diagnose a specific cause of dementia

*These are guidelines on the guidelines and are not meant to be comprehensive

General issues

Treatment of dementia

Depression

Detection

Treatment

Other disorders

Delirium

Schizophrenia

Parkinson's disease

Learning disability

Other guidelines

Organisation of services

Standards of care

Inquiries into care

Carers

Index

208